OXFORD SPECIALTY TRAINING

Long Cases for the Final FRC

OXFORD SPECIALTY TRAINING

Long Cases for the Final FRCR 2B

Dr Rebecca Hanlon DMRD FRCR

Dr John Curtis FRCP DMRD FRCR

Dr Hulya Wieshmann MRCP FRCR

Dr David White DMRD FRCR

Dr Caren Landes MRCPCH FRCR

Dr Val Gough MRCS FRCR FFRRSCI

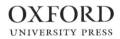

OXFORD
UNIVERSITY PRESS

OXFORD
UNIVERSITY PRESS

Great Clarendon Street, Oxford OX2 6DP

Oxford University Press is a department of the University of Oxford.
It furthers the University's objective of excellence in research, scholarship,
and education by publishing worldwide in

Oxford New York

Auckland   Cape Town   Dar es Salaam   Hong Kong   Karachi
Kuala Lumpur   Madrid   Melbourne   Mexico City   Nairobi
New Delhi   Shanghai   Taipei   Toronto

With offices in

Argentina   Austria   Brazil   Chile   Czech Republic   France   Greece
Guatemala   Hungary   Italy   Japan   Poland   Portugal   Singapore
South Korea   Switzerland   Thailand   Turkey   Ukraine   Vietnam

Oxford is a registered trade mark of Oxford University Press
in the UK and in certain other countries

Published in the United States
by Oxford University Press Inc., New York

British Library Cataloguing in Publication Data
Data available

Library of Congress Cataloging in Publication Data
Data available

Typeset by Glyph International, Bangalore, India
Printed in Great Britain
by
CPI Antony Rowe, Chippenham, Witshire

ISBN 978-0-19-959000-1

10 9 8 7 6 5 4 3 2 1

To our children:

Emily, James, Matthew, Handan, Timothy, Ben,
Andrew, Abigail, Hugo, Eliza, and Niamh

Foreword

The authors have conducted examination preparation courses for many years and are completely aware of the requirements for the FRCR (UK) examinations. They are completely 'up to date' and have chosen excellent cases that match those seen in the examination.

Included in the answers are observations of the radiology signs, interpretation of these signs, the diagnosis, and, where applicable, a differential diagnosis. There are notes on the further management of these cases and, as a 'bonus', extensive key points about the disease which are excellent for revision. The wide range of cases is excellent. The authors have taken into account, and produced cases dealing with, organ radiology, modality topics, age specialisation, and interventional radiology.

This is an excellent test, full of wonderful cases, fun to read, and with masses of information.

Radiologists who have completed their examination can also make use of the book for revision and testing their ongoing skills and knowledge.

This is an absolute MUST for every teaching hospital imaging department.

Professor Philip Gishen
MB, B.ch., DMRD, FRCR
Director of Imaging
Imperial College Healthcare NHS Trust

Contents

Introduction

At the time of writing this book, the written part of the Final FRCR 2B examination consists of a reporting session followed immediately by a rapid reporting session.

The reporting session lasts for 55 minutes during which time you will be expected to report on six cases. This will give you approximately 9 minutes per case. Some cases will be less complex and therefore will be quicker to answer, allowing you a little extra time for the harder cases.

It is essential that you answer all the questions—even if you do not arrive at the exact diagnosis you will be given marks for correct observations/interpretations, a sensible differential diagnosis, and further management.

A short clinical history is provided for each case. It is essential that you read the clinical information carefully and interpret the images according to the clinical scenario. This will help you to narrow your differential diagnosis.

Each case may comprise up to four images or imaging sequences. The images are displayed digitally using a computer workstation. Each candidate has his/her own work station which comprises an Apple Mac Mini, a 19 inch monitor, and a mouse (no keyboard). The images are displayed using Osirix. This allows them to be manipulated in the usual way, i.e. zoom, pan, magnify etc. If possible, make sure that you are familiar with this system before the exam. A short demonstration and some practice cases are provided just before the exam commences so that you can familiarize yourself with the system. You can move through the cases in numerical order, or skip a case and come back to it if you are struggling.

When recording your findings it is essential that the examiner can read your handwriting! If your handwriting is illegible you will not be given credit for a good answer. Ask a friend or colleague to give you their opinion on one of your answers in the run up to the exam. If your reports are well structured, you will give the examiner the impression that you are a clear logical thinker and good radiologist!

You are advised by the Royal College to use a standard format which will aid in structuring your report and help the examiners to mark your answer. In our experience it is much easier to mark answers when subheadings and bullet points or numbers are used. The College advice may change, so always refer to guidance on the website: http://www.rcr.ac.uk/docs/radiology/pdf/CandGuide-Notes-Nov2009.pdf

Reports should be succinct and to the point. Do not list the dates of investigations, imaging sequences, or repeat the clinical information as this will waste valuable time.

Recommended format of report

Observations

In this section, you should write down all relevant positive and negative findings on all the available imaging studies.

Interpretation

Here you should record your interpretation of the findings: for example, whether a bone lesion is benign or malignant and the reason behind your thinking.

Main or principal diagnosis

In this section you should try to come to a single most likely diagnosis. If this is not possible, then state here which diagnosis you feel is most likely and why.

Differential diagnoses

For some cases there will be no differential diagnosis. If there is a list of potential differential diagnoses, keep this brief and list in order of likeliness. Explain why these diagnoses are less likely than the principal diagnosis.

Any relevant further investigations or management

In this section you should suggest any further appropriate investigations or clinical management such as biopsy, discussion at a multidisciplinary meeting, referral to a specialist centre, etc.

Specimen reports are available on the College website. The College has also provided specimen answers where the observations and interpretations are combined under one heading. This is perfectly acceptable and is the format we have used for the answers in this textbook.

Some cases will be straightforward with very little description, differential diagnoses, or further management. Do not feel the need to pad these cases out with extra information if it is not needed, as you may lose marks.

If there is one clear diagnosis, do not give a long list of differential diagnoses. This will detract from a good answer and give the impression that you cannot be decisive. If there is a list of differentials keep this brief and realistic—limited to one or two where possible. You will lose marks for incorrect statements or for showing a lack of discrimination in your conclusions.

In some cases there may be no further management; therefore do not suggest inappropriate investigations. You will lose marks for suggesting tests that are unnecessary, expensive, invasive, or use ionizing radiation inappropriately. It is important to be as realistic as possible with your further management. Think what you would do in day-to-day working practice.

Remember to think about the combination of imaging that the examiners have given you as this can also be a clue to the diagnosis. For example, a small-bowel meal and an HRCT chest would suggest scleroderma.

Look for patterns and common associations, i.e. if you see interstitial fibrosis on a chest X-ray or CT look for an underlying cause by searching for a dilated oesophagus (scleroderma), asbestos plaques (asbestosis), dense liver (amiodarone therapy), or rheumatoid shoulders (rheumatoid lung).

The next part of the 2B exam involves a rapid reporting session which consists of reporting 30 films in 35 minutes. The films are a mixture of normal and abnormal cases and are supposed to simulate an A&E or GP 'reporting pile'. Each case will comprise a single examination but may show multiple images (e.g. AP, oblique, and lateral views of the wrist).

You will be asked to record whether you think the film is normal or abnormal. For those cases that you feel are abnormal, you should briefly describe the abnormality on the pre-printed answer sheet provided. The abnormal finding will require a fairly short description as the 'box' in which to write your answer is relatively small. There is only one abnormality on each film and this will be unequivocally abnormal. It may be on the edge of the film but it will be a definite abnormality.

One of the main reasons for failing the rapid reporting is to overcall normal films. Make sure that you report plenty of plain films in the run-up to the exam to get a feel for normality. It is a good idea to browse through Keats' book of normal variants (Keats and Anderson 2006) just before the exam. One of the reasons for failing the rapid reporting is misinterpretation of normal variants, such as accessory ossicles, ossification centres, and fusing epiphyses, as fractures or age-related changes and anatomical variants should be recorded as 'normal'.

Remember—a good rule of thumb is that if you are taking a while to decide if something is abnormal, then it probably is not! The exam has not been designed to trip you up and the abnormalities will be real, not subtle. Remember to think as a working radiologist and report in the same way as you would when reporting plain films day to day.

Good luck!

Rebecca Hanlon

Reference

Keats TE, Anderson MW. *Atlas of Normal Roentgen Variants That May Simulate Disease* (8th edn). St Louis, MO: Mosby, 2006

Exam 1

Case 1.1

Clinical details

A 66-year-old male with a chronic history of progressive shortness of breath.

Imaging

Figure 1.1a Axial HRCT chest, supine image.
Figure 1.1b Axial HRCT chest, prone image.
Figure 1.1c Axial CT image through mediastinum.
Figure 1.1d Axial CT image through liver, unenhanced.

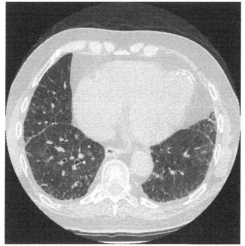

1.1a

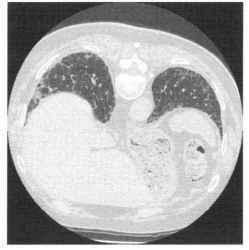

1.1b

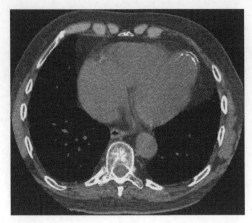

1.1c

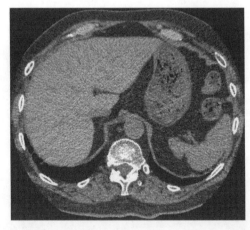

1.1d

Observations and interpretations

- Figure 1.1a shows an image of the lung bases with areas of sub-pleural reticular change, septal thickening, and ground glass shadowing. No effusions.
- Figure 1.1b shows that the sub-pleural changes persist in the prone position with the appearance of sub-pleural crescents.
- Figure1.1c shows cardiomegaly with calcification in the wall of the left ventricle in keeping with a left ventricular aneurysm.
- Figure1.1d shows increased density of the liver relative to the spleen.

Principal diagnosis

- Interstitial pulmonary fibrosis and increased density of the liver secondary to amiodarone treatment.
- The left ventricular aneurysm may be causing a dysrhythmia, therefore requiring treatment with amiodarone.

Differential diagnosis

- Idiopathic pulmonary fibrosis—however, this would not explain the increased density of the liver.

Table 1.1a Differential diagnosis

Causes of basal pulmonary fibrosis	Causes of increased density of the liver on CT
Drug-related • **Amiodarone** • Bleomycin • Busulphan • Nitrofurantoin	Drug-related • **Amiodarone**
Asbestosis	Heavy metal deposition • Gold • Copper • Thorotrast • Thallium • Iron • Iodine
Rheumatoid arthritis	Haemochromatosis
Scleroderma	Glycogen storage diseases
Idiopathic pulmonary fibrosis	Acute massive protein deposits

Further management

- Correlation with clinical history.
- Review previous HRCT scans of the chest to assess progression of basal lung changes.

Key points

- Amiodarone toxicity is seen in 5–10% of patients and develops after a period of 1–12 months of treatment.
- Occurs in 14–18% on long-term therapy.
- The risk is increased with a daily dose >400mg.
- The prognosis is good after discontinuation of the drug.
- Findings on an HRCT scan of the lungs in the acute stage include focal peripheral consolidation. In the chronic stage alveolar and interstitial infiltrates develop with areas of pleural thickening.
- Associated with this is high attenuation of liver (95–145HU) relative to spleen (normal value for liver, 30–70HU).

Table 1.1b What to look for on a chest X-ray in the viva to help differentiate causes of pulmonary fibrosis

Amiodarone
- Dense liver
- Additional signs of cardiac failure: effusions, cardiomegaly, calcified left ventricular aneurysm, pacing wires

Asbestosis
- Calcified pleural plaques
- Rounded atelectasis

Rheumatoid arthritis
- Erosive change in shoulders
- Erosion of ends of clavicles
- Shoulder joint replacement
- Pleural effusions
- Pulmonary nodules ± cavitation *rheumatoid nodules*

Scleroderma
- Dilated oesophagus
- Aspiration pneumonia

Idiopathic pulmonary fibrosis
- Probable diagnosis in the absence of any of the above

References

Akira M, Ishikawa H, Yamamoto S. Drug-induced pneumonitis: thin-section CT findings in 60 patients. *Radiology* **224**: 852–60, 2002

Dähnert W. *Radiology Review Manual* (6th edn). Lippincott–Williams & Wilkins, 2007

Meyer CA, White CS, Sherman KE. Diseases of the hepatopulmonary axis. *Radiographics* **20**: 687–98, 2000

Notes

Case 1.2

Clinical details

A 27-year-old female presenting with tinnitus.

Imaging

Selected MRI images of the brain.

Figure 1.2a Coronal T1W MRI image of the internal auditory meati (IAMS) post-gadolinium
Figures 1.2b–e Selected axial T1W MRI images of the IAMS and brain post-gadolinium

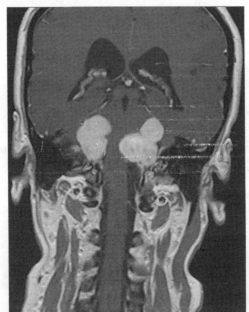

1.2a

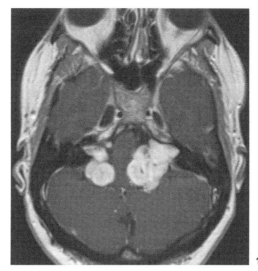

1.2b

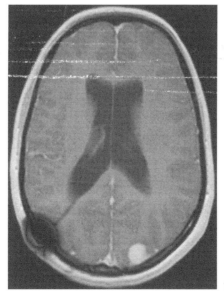

1.2c

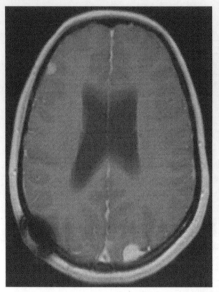 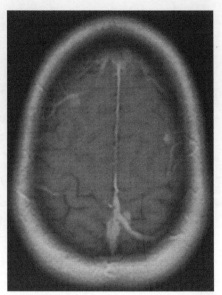

1.2d   1.2e

Observations and interpretations

- Figures 1.2a and 1.2b show large, bilateral cerebellopontine angle lesions which enhance intensely post gadolinium. The masses indent both cerebellopontine angles (CPA) and extend into the internal auditory meati. There is a right ventricular shunt in situ and a degree of hydrocephalus due to obstruction of the fourth ventricle by the bilateral CPA lesions. The appearances are in keeping with bilateral acoustic neuromas.
- Figure 1.2c to e show small, enhancing dural based masses involving the left occipital region, the right frontal region and the vertex. There is no significant mass effect. The appearances would be in keeping with multiple meningiomata.

Principal diagnosis

- Neurofibromatosis type 2 with bilateral acoustic neuromas, and multiple intracranial meningiomata.

Differential diagnosis

- There is no other differential that would give these imaging features.

Table 1.2a Differential diagnosis

CP angle lesion	Meningeal thickening
• Acoustic neuroma	• **Meningioma**
• Facial nerve schwannoma	• Metastasis
• Meningioma	• Sarcoidosis
• Epidermoid cyst	• Non Hodgkins Lymphoma
• Endolymphatic sac tumour	• Infections – TB, fungal
• Metastasis	

Further management

- Neurosurgical referral for consideration of radio surgery to acoustic neuromas
- MRI spine to exclude associated meningiomas, neurofibromata, and cord ependymomas
- Genetic screening

Key points

- Neurofibromatosis type 2 (NF2, central neurofibromatosis) is an inherited autosomal dominant syndrome due to an abnormality of chromosome 22.
- The incidence is 1 in 50,000 and symptoms tend to develop in the second decade of life.
- Characteristic associations are:
  - bilateral acoustic neuromas
  - meningiomas/meningiomatosis
  - gliomas
  - schwannomas of other cranial nerves
  - paraspinal neurofibromas
  - spinal cord ependymomas
  - spinal cord meningiomas.

Reference

Shu RR, Mirowitz SA, Wippold FJ 2nd. Neurofibromatosis; MR imaging findings involving the head and spine. *American Journal of Roentgenology* **160**: 159–64, 2003

Notes

CPA angle tumour
- acoustic neuroma
- meningioma
- epidermoid
- arachnoid cyst
- aneurysm of basilar artery
- choroid plexus papilloma
- glomus jugulare tumour
- metastasis

Case 1.3

Clinical details

A 10-year-old girl presenting with visual disturbance and headaches.

Imaging

Figure 1.3a Axial CT image of the brain—unenhanced.
Figure 1.3b Sagittal MRI image of the brain—T1W post-gadolinium.

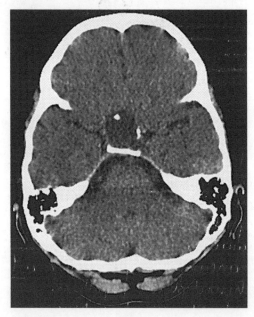

1.3a

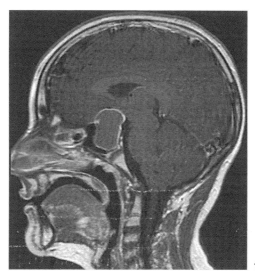

1.3b

Observations and interpretations

- Figure 1.3a shows a cystic mass in the suprasellar region with two areas of peripheral calcification. No significant mass effect or oedema.
- Figure 1.3b again demonstrates a large cystic mass centred on the suprasellar region and extending inferiorly into the sphenoid sinus. There is peripheral enhancement in the wall of the cyst. No significant mass effect or hydrocephalus is demonstrated.

Principal diagnosis

- Craniopharyngioma.

Differential diagnosis *cystic*

- Epidermoid—unlikely because of lack of solid components.
- Rathke's cleft cyst—unlikely because of the calcification.
- Arachnoid cyst—unlikely because of the peripheral enhancement.
- *empty sella*

Further management

- Referral for neurosurgical opinion.

mixed cystic + solid
├ craniopharyngioma –
└ macroadenoma –

Key points

- Craniopharyngiomas are benign tumours originating from epithelial rests along the vestigial craniopharyngeal duct.
- They are the most common cause of a suprasellar mass in children.
- There are two age peaks: in the first to second decade (75%) and in the fifth decade (25%). They are more common in males.
- Clinical presentation is due to the effects of compression of adjacent structures: diabetes insipidus, growth retardation, bitemporal hemianopia, headaches from hydrocephalus.
- They can be intra/suprasellar or ectopic in the floor of the third ventricle or in the sphenoid bone.
- The usual CT appearance is of a cystic suprasellar mass with marginal calcification and peripheral enhancement post-contrast. Calcification is more commonly seen in childhood tumours than in adulthood.
- The tumours may also be completely or partly solid and show enhancement of the solid areas post-contrast.
- On MRI the signal intensity of the cystic component on T1W images is variable depending on the contents of the cysts, i.e. proteinaceous fluid, cholesterol, haemorrhage. The cyst is hyperintense on T2W images and shows peripheral enhancement post-gadolinium.
- The differential diagnosis includes epidermoid, Rathke's cleft cyst, and arachnoid cyst.
- Epidermoids are mixed solid and cystic masses in the suprasellar fossa, where the solid component is larger than the cystic element. They do not typically show peripheral enhancement.
- Rathke's cleft cysts are small intrasellar lesions typically located between the anterior and posterior parts of the pituitary gland. They are not typically calcified.
- Arachnoid cysts are thin-walled cysts containing CSF and do not show enhancement.

References

Dähnert W. *Radiology Review Manual* (6th edn). Lippincott–Williams & Wilkins, 2007.

Donnelly L (ed). *Diagnostic Imaging: Pediatrics.* Amirysys, 2005; **7**: 110–12.

Rossi A, Cama A, Consales A, *et al.* Neuroimaging of pediatric craniopharyngiomas: a pictorial essay. *Journal of Pediatric Endocrinology and Metabolism* **19** (Suppl 1): 299–319, 2006.

Tsuda M, Takahashi S, Higano S, Kurihara N, Ikeda H, Sakamoto K. CT and MR imaging of craniopharyngioma. *European Radiology* **7**: 464–9, 1997.

Notes

Suprasellar mass

- Meningioma ⑦
- Craniopharyngioma ⑧
- Chiasmal + optic nerve glioma ②
- Hypothalamic glioma ③
  - Hamartoma tuber cinerum ④
- Infundibular tumour ⑤
  - glioma
  - lymphoma
  - histiocytosis, sarcoid
- Germinoma (TB) ⑨
- Epidermoid / Dermoid ⑩
- Arachnoid cyst ⑪
- Suprasellar aneurysm ⑥
- Rathke's cleft cyst ⑫
- Pituitary macro-adenoma ①

SATCMO

Sarcoidosis, Sella neoplasm c̄ superior extension
Aneurysm, Arachnoid cyst, Adenoma
Tuberculosis, Teratoma
Craniopharyngioma, Chordoma
Meningioma, Metastatic disease, Mucocele
Optic nerve glioma, neuroma

Hyperintense Suprasellar Mass on T1W]
thrombosed aneurysm, craniopharyngioma, germinoma,
Rathke's cleft cyst, haemorrhagic met, cavernous angioma,
dermoid cyst, lipoma, ectopic neurohypophysis

Case 1.4

Clinical details

A 56-year-old female presenting with progressive right-sided elbow swelling.

Imaging

Figure 1.4a Right elbow—lateral view.
Figure 1.4b Right elbow—AP view.
Figure 1.4c Sagittal T2W MRI—cervical spine.
Figure 1.4d Sagittal T1W MRI—cervical spine.

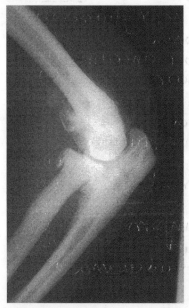 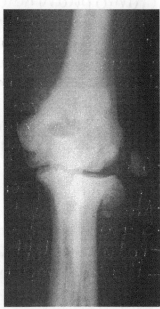

1.4a   1.4b

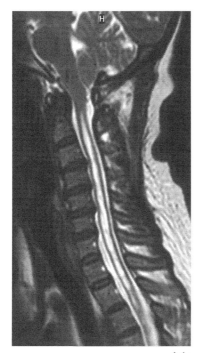
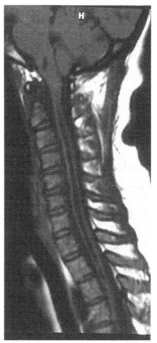

1.4c   1.4d

Observations and interpretations

- Figures 1.4a and 1.4b show gross abnormality of the elbow joint. There is generalized increased density of the visualized bones and a joint effusion. There are several ossific fragments within the elbow joint as well as healed fractures in the distal humerus and radial neck.
- Figures 1.4c and 1.4d show a cavity in the spinal cord from C2 to T3 which is low signal on the T1W image and high signal on the T2W image. The appearances are those of a syrinx of the cervico-thoracic cord.
- There is herniation of the cerebellar tonsils through the foramen magnum with mild compression on the medulla oblongata.

Principal diagnosis

- Syringomyelia with cerebellar herniation. These appearances are compatible with an Arnold Chiari type 1 malformation.
- Neuropathic changes (Charcot's arthropathy) of the right elbow.

Differential diagnosis

- None in this case.

Table 1.4a Differential diagnosis

Cystic lesions in the spinal cord	Increased bone density and disorganized joint space
• Syringomyelia • Myelomalacia • Cystic spinal cord tumour, astrocytoma, haemangioblastoma • Ventriculus terminalis (normal variant)	• Neuropathic joint

Table 1.4b Differential diagnosis

Causes of a neuropathic joint	Causes of a syrinx
• Syringomyelia • Syphilis • Diabetes mellitus • Leprosy • Congenital insensitivity to pain • Frostbite	• Post-traumatic • Post-inflammatory: infection, surgery, post subarachnoid haemorrhage, myelitis • Tumour associated • Ischaemia

Table 1.4c Neuropathic joint '5Ds'

- Dense subchondral bone
- Destruction of articular cortex
- Deformity
- Debris
- Dislocation

Further management

- Post intravenous gadolinium images of the spinal cord are required to exclude a cord tumour which may be associated with the syrinx.
- Neurosurgical follow-up.

Key points

- Arnold–Chiari type 1 is associated with syringomyelia in 75% of cases.
- Normal position of fourth ventricle.
- Associated with skeletal occipito-vertebral anomalies such as basilar impression, occipitalization of the atlas, and Klippel–Feil syndrome.
- Hydrocephalus found in about 40% of cases.
- Arnold–Chiari type 1 malformations—herniation of the cerebellar tonsils >3mm below the foramen magnum.
- Obstruction of the flow of CSF at the foramen magnum leads to syrinx formation within the cord.
- Syringomyelia results in dissociated sensory loss which can cause a neuropathic arthropathy in the joints of the upper limb.
- Repeated trauma of these joints, especially the elbow and shoulder joints, leads to fractures, often healing with exuberant callus, disorganization, and debris—neuropathic (Charcot's) arthropathy.

References

Jones EA, Manaster BJ, May DA, Disler DG. Neuropathic osteoarthropathy: diagnostic dilemmas and differential diagnosis. *Radiographics* **20**: S279–93, 2000.

Poe LB, Coleman LL, and Mahmud, F. Congenital central nervous system anomalies. *Radiographics* **9**: 801–26, 1989.

Images donated by Dr Andrew Smethurst, University Hospital Aintree

Notes

Intramedullary mass: Ependymoma

Tumour — Primary — Astrocytoma, Dermoid, Haemangioblastoma

Secondary — Metastases

Inflammation — Demyelination, Sarcoid, Acute transverse myelitis

Infarct

Haematoma

Syringomyelia — Post traumatic, post-inflammatory, Tumour associated, Ischaemia, Chiari I

Case 1.5

Clinical details

A 19-year-old male presenting with right leg pain.

Imaging

Figure 1.5a AP x-ray of the right knee.
Figure 1.5b Lateral x-ray of the right knee.
Figure 1.5c Whole-body ^{99m}Tc MDP bone scan.

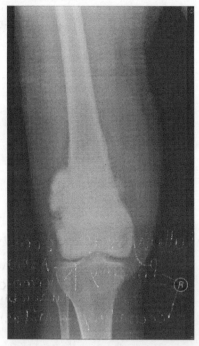

1.5a

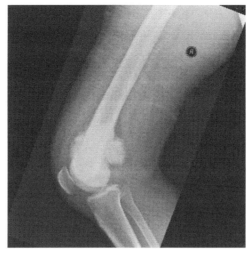

1.5b

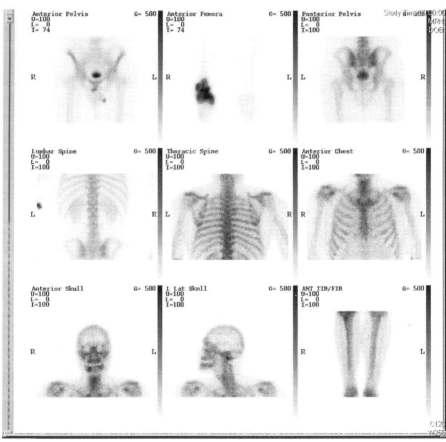

1.5c

Observations and interpretations

- Figures 1.5a and 1.5b show a dense area of sclerosis involving the distal femoral diametaphysis with a wide zone of transition. There is a solid agressive periosteal reaction along the medial and lateral aspect of the distal femoral shaft, and adjacent cloud-like extra osseous masses. There is overlying soft tissue swelling.
- Figure 1.5a shows a solitary intense area of increased tracer activity in the distal femur, no abnormal tracer activity elsewhere to indicate metastatic spread, and no soft tissue uptake in the lungs to indicate pulmonary metastases.

Principal diagnosis

- Osteosarcoma

Differential diagnosis

- Osteomyelitis
- Ewing's sarcoma
- Lymphoma

Table 1.5a Differential diagnosis

Bone sclerosis with periosteal reaction	Differentiating factors from osteosarcoma
Traumatic • Healing fracture	• Radiograph with previous fracture/trauma • Old fracture on plain film
Neoplastic • Metastatic	• History of primary cancer • Axial skeleton affected more commonly than appendicular skeleton • Multiple • Unusual to get a large soft tissue component compared with osteosarcoma
• Lymphoma	• Diaphysis is favoured by lymphoma
• Ewing's sarcoma	• Younger age (5–15 years) • Diaphysis or marrow-rich sites such as pelvis and ribs • 'Onion peel': multi-laminar periosteal reaction resulting from periodic activity • Saucerization: subperiosteal mass may cause erosion of the outer cortex • Can be indistinguishable from osteosarcoma
• Osteoid osteoma	• Well-defined lytic lesions <1cm at centre of smooth eccentric sclerosis
Infective	• Readily crosses the physis • Sequestrum and involucrum • Can be very difficult to differentiate from osteosarcoma

Further management

- MRI of the entire bone to include the joint above and below the tumour.
- Staging CT thorax, abdomen, and pelvis.
- Referral to a bone cancer treatment centre for biopsy and definitive treatment. (Biopsy without knowledge of the operation field may lead to malignant seeding in a non-operative site.)

Key points

radiation

2° { malignant degeneration Paget's

- M:F = 2:1.
- Peak age 10–25 years. Predominantly affects the metaphysis of tubular bones in this age group.
- Second peak in seventh decade.
- May arise in previously irradiated site.
- Presents with pain, mass, and fever. May have mildly elevated alkaline phosphatase. 25% have diabetes mellitus (paraneoplastic).
- Common sites:
  - femur 40% (75% of which around the knee)
  - tibia 15%
  - humerus 15%.
- Imaging features: ill defined mixed sclerotic and lytic areas, or predominantly sclerotic medullary lesions.
- Wide zone of transition.
- Florid 'sunray' periosteal reaction (following Sharpey's fibres). This is characteristic of osteosarcoma but is not specific. In Ewing's sarcoma fibres tend to be fewer and more delicate.
- Codman's triangle.
- 'Cloud-like' matrix of extra-osseous spreading soft tissue mass.
- The open growth plate forms a relative barrier to neoplastic spread. Infection more readily crosses the growth plate.
- 'Skip lesions' are uncommon.
- Haematogenous spread to lungs (predominately subpleural), leading to an increased incidence of pneumothoraces. Metastases to the lungs contain osteoid and have increased tracer activity on bone isotopes.
- Some unusual types of osteosarcoma.
  - Parosteal osteosarcomas (5%). Affect third and fourth decades. Radiologically appear as a dense apparently mature matrix enveloping the shaft, with a well-defined lucency separating the tumour from the normal cortex.
  - Telangiectatic (5%). Thin septations within blood-filled cavities. Pathological fracture is common. Diaphyseal more than metaphyseal. Fluid–fluid level on cross-sectional imaging.

References

Chapman S, Nakielny R. Aids to Radiological Differential Diagnosis (5th edn). Saunders, 2009
Grainger RG, Allison DJ, Adam A, Dixon AK (eds). Grainger & Allison's Diagnostic Radiology: A Textbook of Medical Imaging (4th edn). Churchill Livingstone, 2001

Notes

Case 1.6

Clinical details

A 35-year-old female presenting with acute right upper quadrant pain and collapse in the third trimester of pregnancy.

Imaging

Figures 1.6a–c Axial CT scans through the lower chest/abdomen.

Figure 1.6d Coronal CT scan of the abdomen/pelvis.

Figure 1.6e–f Axial CT scans through the pelvis.

Figure 1.6g Axial T1W MRI of the upper abdomen.

Figure 1.6h T2W fat-suppressed MRI of the upper abdomen.

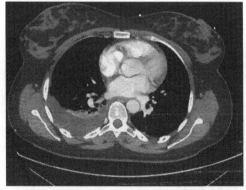

1.6a

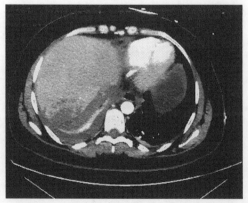

1.6b

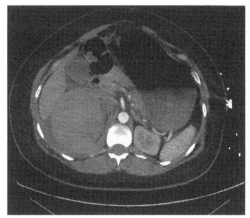

1.6c

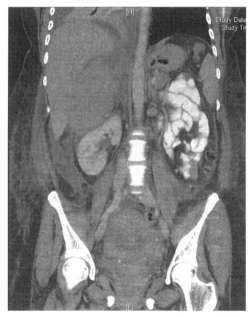

1.6d

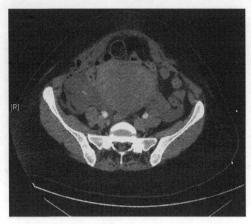

1.6e

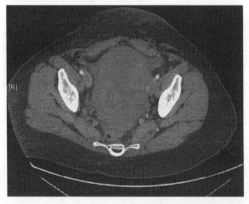

1.6f

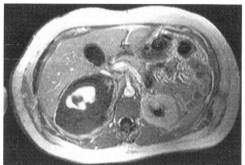

1.6g

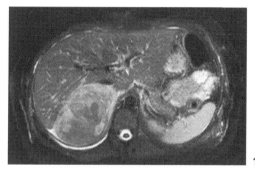

1.6h

Observations and interpretations

- Figure 1.6a shows a large right-sided pleural effusion.
- Figure 1.6b again shows the right pleural effusion posterior to a band of atelectasis at the right lung base. Anterior to the atelectasis is further fluid which is subcapsular in location. There is a focal area of low attenuation in the posterior aspect of the right lobe of the liver (segment 7).
- Figures 1.6c and 1.6d show a large right retroperitoneal mass displacing the kidney inferiorly. The mass is high in attenuation. There is also free fluid laterally in the right side of the abdomen.
- Figures 1.6e and 1.6f show a large post-partum uterus and free fluid in the right side of the abdomen. There is gas in the anterior pelvic wall in keeping with a recent Caesarean section.
- The right retroperitoneal mass is mixed attenuation on the fat-suppressed image (Figure 1.6h) and shows central high signal on the T1W image (Figure 1.6g) in keeping with acute blood.

Principal diagnosis

- HELLP (Haemolysis, elevated liver enzymes, low platelets) syndrome with intraparenchymal and subcapsular haematoma in and around the liver.
- There has been a recent Caesarean section.
- The right retroperitoneal mass is likely to represent an adrenal haemorrhage secondary to low platelets and disseminated intravascular coagulation.

Differential diagnosis

- Haemorrhage from an intra-hepatic tumour such as an adenoma.

Further management

- Supportive management.
- Consider hepatic embolization if bleeding continues.

Key points

- HELLP syndrome stands for haemolysis, elevated liver enzymes, low platelets, and is a severe variant of pre-eclampsia.
- Characterized by subcapsular or intraparenchymal haemorrhage on imaging.
- Usually occurs in primigravidas and before birth in the third trimester. Rare in multiparous women. More common in black females in the second and third decades.
- Occasionally occurs immediately post-partum.
- Findings on CT include acute intraparenchymal haematoma in the liver with areas of increased attenuation in the first 24–72 hours, which become hypodense later. Occasionally active areas of contrast extravasation may be seen in the haematomas.
- Wedge-shaped areas of liver infarction also occur.
- Findings on MRI are variable owing to age of the haematoma and the presence of infarcts.
- Clinical presenatation is with acute right upper quadrant/epigastric pain, signs of pre-eclampsia (i.e. proteinuria, hypertension, and oedema), or eclampsia with convulsions and coma.
- Hb is normally <11g/dl, bilirubin >1.2mg/dl, and platelets <100,000/mm3.
- Complications include hepatic necrosis, rupture of hepatic haematoma with haemoperitoneum, disseminated intravascular coagulation (DIC), abruptio placenta, renal failure, and pulmonary oedema.
- Treatment is supportive: emergency Caesarean section, surgery, or embolization for hepatic bleeding.

References

Federle M, Jeffrey RB, Anne VS. *Diagnostic Imaging: Abdominal*. Amirsys, 2004
Lubner M, Menias C, Rucker C, *et al*. Blood in the belly: CT findings of hemoperitoneum. *Radiographics* **27**: 109–25, 2007

Notes

Exam 2

Case 2.1

Clinical details

A 22-year-old male presenting to accident and emergency following minor facial trauma.

Imaging

Figure 2.1a Orthopantomogram (OPG) X-ray.
Figure 2.1b Axial CT image of the mandible.
Figure 2.1c Whole-body ^{99m}Tc-MDP bone scan.
Figure 2.1d Axial HRCT images of the lungs.

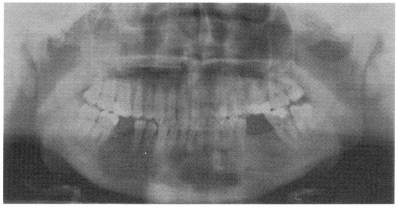

2.1a

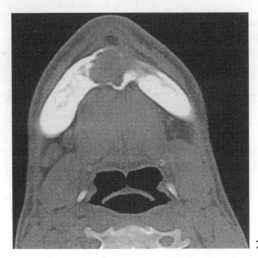

2.1b

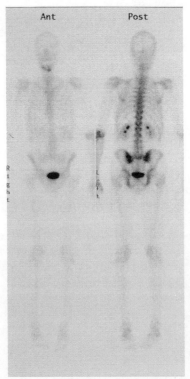

2.1c

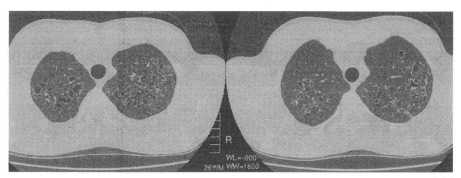

2.1d

Observations and interpretations

- Figure 2.1a shows a lucent lesion in the midline of the mandible. No obvious fracture shown.
- Figure 2.1b shows that the mandibular lesion is well defined and slightly expansile. There is cortical thinning and breakthrough. No overlying soft tissue mass. No fracture demonstrated on CT.
- Figure 2.1c shows increased tracer uptake within the mandibular lesion and normal uptake within the rest of the bony skeleton.
- Figure 2.1d show small nodules and thin-walled cysts in both upper lobes of the lungs. No
✱ pneumothorax.

Principal diagnosis

- Langerhans cell histiocytosis—eosinophilic granuloma in the mandible and multiple pulmonary cysts.

Differential diagnosis

- None in this case.

Table 2.1a Differential diagnosis

Causes of a well-defined lucent lesion in the mandible	Causes of multiple cystic areas in the lungs
- Eosinophilic granuloma - Multiple myeloma—cold on bone scan, multiple lesions - Fibrous dysplasia—ground glass appearance - Radicular cyst—around the tooth apex - Dentigerous cyst—related to the crown of an unerupted tooth. - Ameloblastoma—more common around the angle of the jaw - Brown tumours—hyperparathyroidism - Aneurysmal bone cyst - Giant cell tumour - Haemangioma - Simple bone cyst	- Langerhans cell histiocytosis - Neurofibromatosis - Lymphangiomyomatosis - Tuberous sclerosis - Honeycomb lung—endstage pulmonary fibrosis - Cystic bronchiectasis - Sarcoidosis

Odontogenic keratocyst
↳ multiple → Gorlin-Goltz Syndrome

Further management

- No further radiological management.
- Referral for specialist chest and maxillofacial opinion.

Key points

- Eosinophilic granuloma is the most benign variety of histiocytosis X or Langerhans cell histiocytosis.
- M:F = 3:2.
- Most cases occur in childhood or in young adults with a peak age range of 5–10 years.
- The bone lesions contain histiocytes, eosinophils, and other inflammatory cells. There is an associated blood eosinophilia.

- Bone lesions are solitary in 50–75% and involve (in order of decreasing frequency) the skull, mandible, spine, ribs, and long bones. The lesions are typically well defined, 'punched out', and expansile. There may be an overlying soft tissue mass.
- Lung involvement primarily affects cigarette smokers.
- There is peribronchiolar proliferation of Langerhans cell infiltrates that form small nodules ranging from 5 to 10mm in size with a predilection for the upper and middle lobes of the lungs. The nodular lesions frequently cavitate and form thick- and thin-walled cysts. These are thought to represent enlarged airway lumina. Pneumothorax due to rupture of the cysts is a recognized complication. In chronic cases there are reticulonodular changes in the mid to upper zones of the lungs.
- The radiological abnormalities may regress, resolve completely, become stable, or progress to advanced cystic changes.
- Treatment consists of smoking cessation, but corticosteroid therapy may be useful in selected patients. Chemotherapeutic agents and lung transplantation may be offered to patients with advanced disease.
- The prognosis of the lung involvement is variable. There may be spontaneous regression, stabiliza-tion, or recurrence of disease.

References

Abbott GF, Melissa L. Rosado-de-Christenson ML, Franks TJ, Frazier AA, Galvin JR. From the archives of the AFIP: pulmonary Langerhans cell histiocytosis. *Radiographics* **24**: 821–41, 2004

Dähnert W. *Radiology Review Manual* (6th edn). Lippincott–Williams & Wilkins, 2007

Notes

Radiolucent lesion of manible.
- periapical cyst
- dentigerous cyst [containing crown of unerupted tooth]
- odontogenic kefatocyst [unilocular]
- ameloblastoma [multilocutated expansile "soap-bubble"]
- giant cell tumour
- haemangioma
- aneurysmal bone cyst
- solitary bone cyst
- eosinophilic granuloma
- multiple myeloma
- fibrous dysplasia
- browns tumour [loss of lamina dura around teeth]

Case 2.2

Clinical details

A 35-year-old male patient presenting with headaches and imbalance.

Imaging

Figures 2.2a–b Sagittal T1W MRI brain pre- and post-gadolinium.
Figures 2.2c–d Axial T1W MRI brain pre- and post-gadolinium.
Figures 2.2e–f Coronal T2W MRI of the upper abdomen.
Figure 2.2g Axial T2W MRI through the upper pole of the kidneys.
Figures 2.2h–i Axial fat-suppressed MRI images of the upper abdomen.

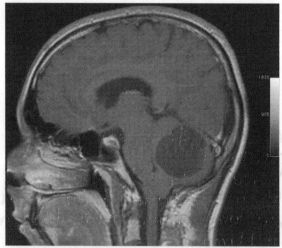

2.2a

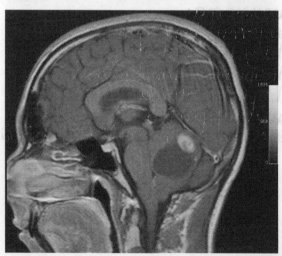

2.2b

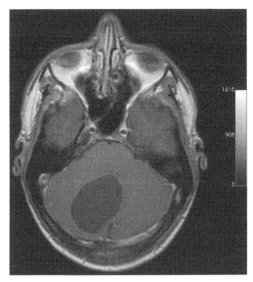

2.2c

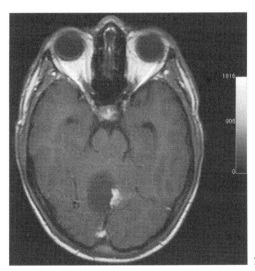

2.2d

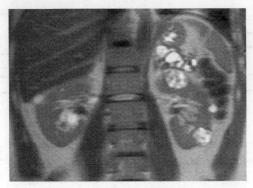

2.2e

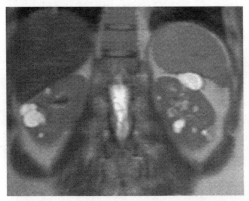

2.2f

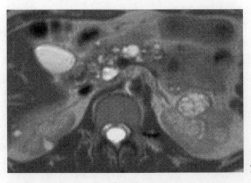

2.2g

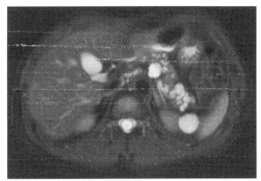

2.2h

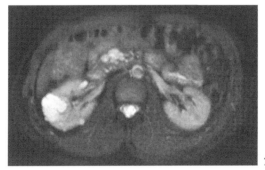

2.2i

Observations and interpretations

- Figures 2.2a–2.2d show a midline cystic lesion in the right cerebellar hemisphere compressing the fourth ventricle. Post-gadolinium there is a nodule of enhancement in the wall of the cyst. The appearances are in keeping with a cystic neoplasm with a mural nodule.
- Figures 2.2e–2.2g show multiple simple cysts in both kidneys. In addition, there are two complex cystic masses in the left kidney—one in the upper and one in the lower pole. These show internal solid elements and a surrounding low signal capsule suggesting renal neoplasms.
- Figures 2.2h and 2.2i show multiple simple-looking cysts in the pancreas.

Principal diagnosis

- Von Hippel–Lindau (VHL) syndrome comprising a cerebellar haemangioblastoma, pancreatic and renal cysts, and two solid renal masses in the left kidney likely to be renal cell carcinomas.

Differential diagnosis

- The appearances of the brain, pancreas, and kidneys point to a diagnosis of VHL with no real differential diagnosis.

Table 2.2a Differential diagnosis

Cystic posterior fossa mass	Pancreatic cysts	Renal cysts
• Haemangioblastoma • Astrocytoma • Metastasis • Lateral medulloblastoma • Choroid plexus papilloma	• VHL • Pseudocyst • Cystadenoma/carcinoma • Intraductal papillary mucinous tumour (IPMT) • Congenital cyst • Adult polycystic kidney disease • Retention cyst	• VHL • Simple cyst • Renal cell carcinoma • Adult polycystic kidney disease • Abscess

Further management

- MRI of the whole spine to exclude further haemangioblastomas.
- Referral to a neurological multidisciplinary team (MDT) to discuss surgical resection of the cerebellar haemangioblastoma.
- Referral to a urology MDT for discussion of partial nephrectomy or radiofrequency ablation/ further staging of the renal cell carcinomas.
- Genetic testing to identify a deletion or significant mutation to confirm the diagnosis.
- Screening of family members.

Key points

- Features of VHL
  - CNS—retinal angiomatosis (von Hippel–Lindau tumour) is the earliest manifestation of the disease and is seen in over 45% of cases, haemangioblastomas (cerebellum, brainstem, spinal cord, retina), endolymphatic sac tumours.
  - Pancreas—cysts, cystadenoma/carcinoma, haemangioblastoma, islet cell tumours.

- ◆ Kidneys—cysts, renal cell carcinoma, adenoma, haemangioma.
- ◆ Adrenal—phaeochromocytoma.
- ◆ Epididymis—cystadenoma.
- ◆ Liver—haemangioma, adenoma.
- Autosomal dominant.
- Age at onset 20–30 years.
- Median life expectancy is 49 years.
- The most common cause of death is from complications of cerebellar haemangioblastomas. The second most common causes are renal cell carcinomas and a broad spectrum of manifestations of the disease.
- Renal tumours occur at a younger age in VHL—mean age is in the early thirties. Annual screening of kidneys by ultrasound is advised to detect malignant transformation of renal cysts.
- Renal cell carcinoma is seen in 20–45% of cases. It may be multifocal, bilateral, and arise in a cyst wall. Renal cell carcinoma is the cause of death in 30–50% of cases; 50% have metastases at the time of discovery.
- Benign pancreatic cysts are usually asymptomatic, do not progress, and are managed conservatively.
- CNS involvement usually precedes the onset of renal disease.
- CNS haemangioblastomas are the most common manifestation of VHL Lesions may be solid, cystic, or haemorrhagic. When cystic they typically have an enhancing mural nodule.
- Treatment is surgical resection or stereotactic radiosurgical ablation.
- Preoperative arterial embolization for extensive spinal cord tumours can also be performed.

References

Choyke PL, Glenn GM, Walther MM, Patronas MJ, Linehan WM, Zbar B. von Hippel–Lindau disease: genetic, clinical and imaging features. *Radiology* 194: 629–42, 1995

Leung RS, Biswas SV, Duncan M, Rankin S. Imaging features of von Hippel–Lindau disease. *Radiographics* 28: 65–79, 2008

Notes

Von Hippel–Lindau (AD)
CNS age 25-35
- retinal angiomatosis
- haemangioblastomas CNS
Heart
└ rhabdomyoma
Kidneys
- cortical renal cysts
- RCC
- renal adenoma
- renal haemangioma
Adrenal
phaeochromocytoma.
Pancreas - pancreatic cystadenoma
└ pancreatic cyst
└ pancreatic islet tumour
└ pancreatic haemangioblastoma.

Case 2.3

Clinical details

A 19-month-old girl presenting with anorexia and abdominal swelling.

Imaging

Figures 2.3a–b Selected axial CT scans of the abdomen post-contrast.
Figure 2.3c Wholebody [¹³¹I]meta-iodobenzylguanidine (MIBG) scan.

↳medullary disease

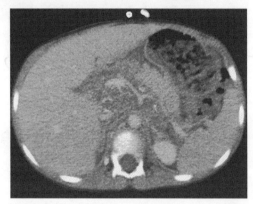

2.3a

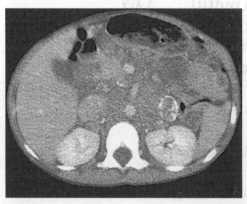

2.3b

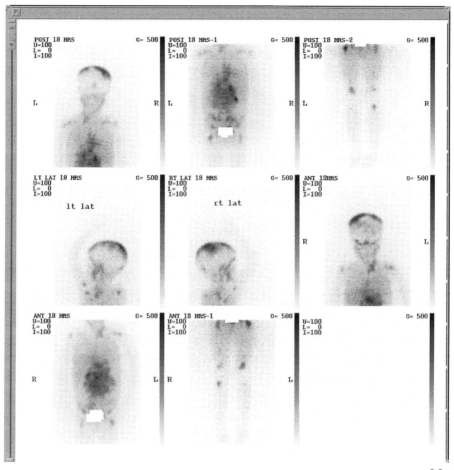

2.3c

Observations and interpretations

- Figure 3.3a shows abnormal soft tissue centred on the retroperitoneum encasing the aorta, coeliac axis, and superior mesenteric artery. The soft tissue extends to the porta hepatis and is separate from the kidneys.
- Figure 3.3b shows a rounded area of calcification within the soft tissue anterior to the left kidney. There is a further rounded soft tissue mass anterior to the right kidney which could arise in the right adrenal. No focal liver lesions as far as seen.
- Figure 3.3c shows abnormal uptake of MIBG in the region of the retroperitoneal mass. There are also focal areas of uptake in the skull, pelvis, right posterior ribs, left clavicle, both femora, both humeral heads, and both proximal tibiae in keeping with bone metastases.

Principal diagnosis

- Metastatic neuroblastoma.

Differential diagnosis

- Wilms' tumour is less likely as the kidneys are not involved on these images. Wilms' tumour displaces vessels rather than encasing them and does not commonly calcify.

Table 2.3a Differential diagnosis

Neuroblastoma	Wilms' tumour
• Peak age <2 years	• Peak age 3 years
• Calcification seen in 75%	• Calcification seen in 10%
• Commonly encases vessels and extends across the midline	• Arises from kidney and displaces adjacent structures but does not cross midline
• Rarely invades vessels	• Associated with invasion of the ipsilateral renal vein and IVC
• Metastasizes to bone and liver	• Metastasizes to lung

Further management

- Review CT images of the lungs and liver to complete the staging.
- MRI scan of the brain.
- Referral to specialist paediatric oncology MDT to discuss treatment options.

Key points

1/3 other site

- Neuroblastoma is the most common abdominal malignancy in infancy.
- M:F 1:1.
- Peak age is at 2 years

1/3 adrenal 1/3 retroperitoneal

- Arises from primitive neural crest. A third are adrenal in location, a third are extra-adrenal in the retroperitoneum, and a third arise at other sites, i.e within the sympathetic neural chain in the neck, mediastinum, retroperitoneum, or pelvis.
- There is a wide clinical presentation including pain, fever, abdominal pain, abdominal mass, bone pain, limp, inability to walk, intractable diarrhoea due to raised vasoactive intestinal polypeptides (VIPs).

- Increased catecholamine production can result in hypertension, flushing, tachycardia, headaches, and acute cerebellar encephalopathy.
- Bone metastases occur in 60% and are typically lytic.
- Metastatic spread also occurs to regional lymph nodes, liver, brain, dura, maxillofacial region, orbits, and lungs.
- The appearance on CT is usually of a large supra-renal mass of mixed attenuation due to areas of haemorrhage, necrosis, and calcification.
- There may be invasion of adjacent structures such as the kidneys, liver, and the spinal canal through the neural foramina.
- Contiguous retroperitoneal lymphadenopathy is seen in >70%.
- The prognosis is better if the age of onset is less than 1 year rather than over 1 year.

References

Dähnert W. *Radiology Review Manual* (5th edn). Lippincott–Williams & Wilkins, 2005

Donnelly L (ed). *Diagnostic Imaging: Pediatrics*. Amirysys, 2005; **5**: 78–80

McHugh K. Renal and adrenal tumours in children. *Cancer Imaging* **7**: 41–51, 2007

Notes

Association

- Beckwith-Wiedemann
- DiGeorge syndrome
- Hischsprung disease
- NF type I

Accompanying syndromes

Hutchinson syndrome
Pepper syndrome — hepatomegaly
Blueberry muffin syndrome — multiple cutaneous lesions

MIBG → medullary disease

Bone scan → cortically based disease.

Case 2.4

Clinical details

A 40-year-old male presenting with left wrist swelling after minor trauma.

Imaging

Figure 2.4a X-ray of both hands and wrists.
Figure 2.4b DP, oblique, and lateral view of left wrist.
Figure 2.4c Coronal T1W MRI of the left wrist, unenhanced.
Figure 2.4d Coronal T1W MRI of the left wrist post IV gadolinium.
Figure 2.4e Axial T1W MRI image of the left wrist post IV gadolinium.
Figure 2.4f Axial CT image of the chest—mediastinal windows.
Figure 2.4g Axial CT image of the chest—lung windows.

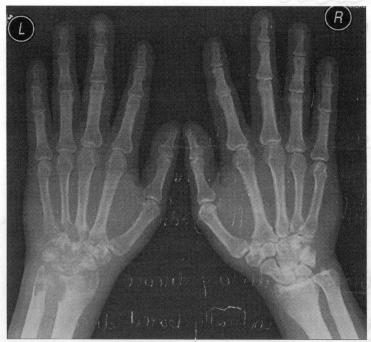

2.4a

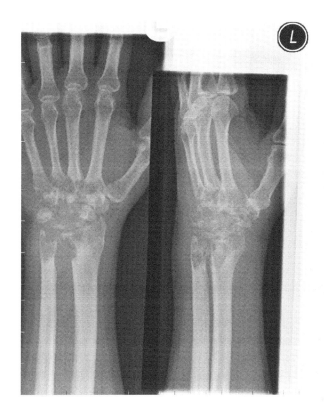

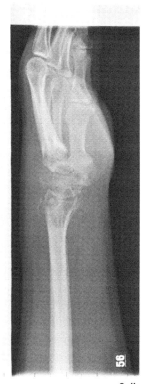

2.4b

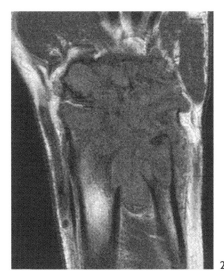

2.4c

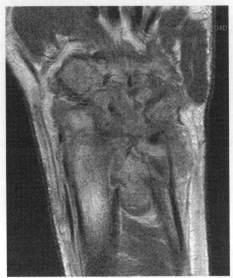

2.4d

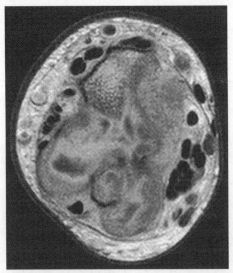

2.4e

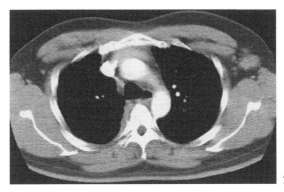

2.4f

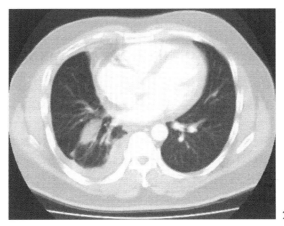

2.4g

Observations and interpretations

- Figures 2.4a and 2.4b show marked destructive change in the intercarpal, radiocarpal, and carpometacarpal joints. There is periarticular osteopenia. The metacarpophalangeal and inter-phalangeal joints are spared. No marked soft tissue swelling or loss of alignment. No periosteal reaction. The contralateral hand and wrist are normal.
- Figures 2.4c and 2.4e show an inflammatory soft tissue mass involving the intercarpal, radiocarpal, and carpometacarpal joints. There is marked enhancement after gadolinium with underlying enhancing pockets of fluid. There is disruption of the interosseous membrane.
- Figures 2.4f and 2.4g show left axillary lymphadenopathy and a right pleural effusion with encysted fluid in the right oblique fissure.

Principal diagnosis

- Destructive arthritis affecting the wrist with penetration of the interosseous membrane likely to be infective.
- Right pleural effusion and left axillary lymphadenopathy makes TB the most likely diagnosis.

Differential diagnosis

- Synovitis of any other cause—unilateral distribution makes infection most likely.
- Rheumatoid arthritis is less likely because of marked destruction and asymmetry.
- Synovial sarcoma is rare and less likely because of the extension across the interosseous membrane—this suggests an infective process.

Table 2.4a Differential diagnosis

Causes of a synovitis	Causes of a pleural effusion	Causes of axillary lymphadenopathy
• Infective: TB • Rheumatoid arthritis • Pigmented villonodular synovitis	• Infective: TB • Collagen vascular diseases: rheumatoid arthritis • Malignant • Vascular: pulmonary embolism • Heart failure • Hypoproteinaemia • Secondary to abdominal disease, i.e. pancreatitis, ascites • Trauma • Miscellaneous: sarcoidosis	• TB • Rheumatoid arthritis • Sarcoidosis • Metastatic • Lymphoma

Further management

- Needle aspiration of fluid in the soft tissue mass under ultrasound guidance.
- Consider image-guided synovial biopsy.

Key points

- Joint involvement by tuberculosis (TB) is usually secondary to adjacent osteomyelitis. TB of the bone is usually secondary to haematogenous spread from primary infection in the lung.
- Occurs in 3–5% of TB patients and in 30% of patients with extrapulmonary TB.

- May be insidious in onset, presenting with chronic pain and disuse.
- More common in middle-aged/elderly patients.
- More common in the hip and knee joints than in the wrist and hand.
- Pannus formation within the joint leads to slow cartilage destruction. Cartilage destruction occurs much more quickly in pyogenic infections.
- Joint space narrowing occurs over several months.
- Juxta-articular osteopenia occurs early, mainly in weight-bearing joints. No marked periosteal reaction compared with pyogenic infections.
- Soft tissues appear normal in the early phase. Later, soft tissue calcification occurs in the healing phase.

References

Dähnert W. *Radiology Review Manual* (6th edn). Lippincott–Williams & Wilkins, 2007

Harisinghani MG, McLoud TC, Shepard JO, Ko JP, Shroff MM, Mueller PR. Tuberculosis from head to toe. *Radiographics* **20**: 449–70, 2000

Hong SH, Kim SM, Ahn JM, Chung HW, Shin MJ, Kang HS. Tuberculous versus pyogenic arthritis: MR imaging evaluation. *Radiology* **218**: 848–53, 2001

Notes

Case 2.5

Clinical details

Routine follow-up of a 37-year-old male with deformity of the right hand and shoulder.

Imaging

Figures 2.5a–b X-ray of right hand including the wrist.
Figure 2.5c X-ray of right shoulder.

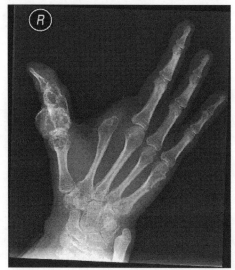

2.5a

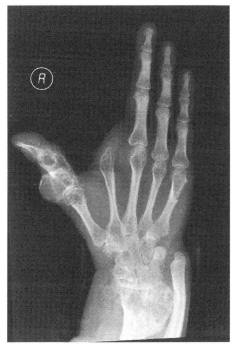

2.5b

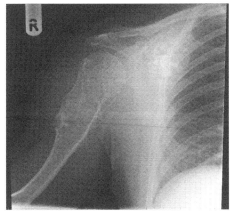

2.5c

Observations and interpretations

- Figures 2.5a and 2.5b show the following:
  - Multiple well-defined expansile lesions involving the head of the first metacarpal, the proximal phalanx of the thumb, and the metaphysis of the distal radius, in keeping with multiple enchondromata.
  - Two small bony spurs arising from the shaft of the fifth metacarpal pointing towards the fifth metacarpophalyngeal joint, in keeping with small osteochondromata. No associated calcification.
  - Discrepancy in length between the radius and ulna, in keeping with a Madelung deformity.
  - No destruction of the bone or aggressive features to suggest malignant transformation.
  - Amputation of the right index finger which may have been as a result of chondrosarcomatous change, debilitating deformity leading to decreased function, or a non-healing pathological fracture.
  - No soft tissue calcification/phleboliths to suggest associated haemangiomas.
- Figure 2.5c shows the following:
  - Expansile lesions arising from the scapula with stippled/focal areas of calcification, in keeping with osteochondromata.
  - Foreshortening of the humerus. Multiple bony exostoses arising from the humeral metaphysis and pointing towards the glenohumeral joint, in keeping with osteochondromata.

Principal diagnosis

- Metachondromatosis

Differential diagnosis

- Ollier's disease—multiple enchondromata, which are usually unilateral as in this case, are seen. However, osteochondromata are not a feature.
- Maffucci's syndrome—multiple enchondromata are seen. However, in this case there are no associated phleboliths/haemangiomas. Osteochondromata are not a feature of Maffucci's syndrome.
- Diaphyseal aclasia—this has multiple ostechondromata and a Madelung deformity but does not have enchondromata.

Table 2.5a Differential diagnosis of multiple cartilaginous lesions

Multiple osteochondromata	Multiple enchondromata
- **Metachondromatosis** - Diaphyseal aclasia	- **Metachondromatosis** - Ollier's disease - Maffucci's syndrome

Further management

- Referral for genetic screening/counselling. Metachondromatosis is transmitted in an autosomal dominant fashion, whereas Ollier's disease and Maffucci's syndrome are non-familial and spontaneous.
- Close clinical observation and appropriate imaging if there is pain, as this may indicate pathological fracture or chondrosarcomatous change.

Key points

- Ollier's disease
  - Synonymous with dyschondroplasia and multiple enchondromatosis.
  - Unilateral predilection.
  - Non-hereditary.
  - Early childhood presentation.
  - Multiple enchondromata predominantly affecting the small bones of the hands and feet.
  - Chondrosarcomatous change and pathological fractures.
- Maffucci's syndrome
  - Features are those of Ollier's disease with soft tissue haemangiomas.
  - Increased prevalence of ovarian carcinoma, pancreatic carcinoma, and gastrointestinal adenocarcinoma.
  - Increased risk of chondrosarcomatous change (30%).
  - Vascular tumours (haemangiosarcomas, lymphangiosarcomas) may develop in a small number of patients.
- Metachondromatosis
  - Autosomal dominant.
  - Combination of multiple osteochondromata and multiple enchondromata.
  - Exostoses point towards the joints (as distinct to diaphyseal aclasia where they point away from the joint space).
- Diaphyseal aclasia
  - Synonymous with multiple osteochondromata, aclasia, familial osteochondromatosis.
  - Autosomal dominant with incomplete penetrance.
  - Metaphysis of long bones. Distance to epiphyseal line increases with growth.
  - Pseudo-Madelung deformity.
  - Short fourth and fifth metacarpals.
  - Coxa vara (25%).
  - Genu valgus (20–40%).
  - Erlenmeyer flask deformity.

References
Kennedy LA. Metachondromatosis. *Radiology* **148**: 117–18, 1983

Notes

Case 2.6

Clinical details

A 58-year-old male patient presenting with flushing and diarrhorrea.

Imaging

Figures 2.6a–d Axial CT images through the upper abdomen and liver.

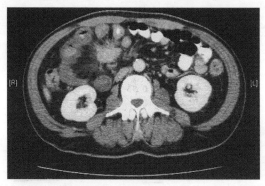

2.6a

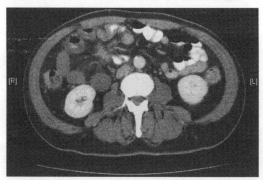

2.6b

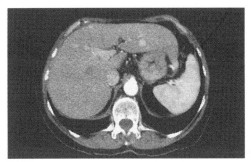

2.6c

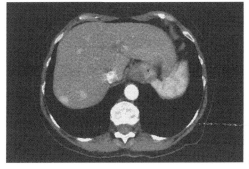

2.6d

Observations and interpretations

- Figures 2.6a and 2.6b show a soft tissue mass in the mesentery in the right upper quadrant of the abdomen. There is a stellate appearance to the surrounding fat, in keeping with a desmoplastic reaction. Surrounding this are several thick-walled loops of small bowel.
- Figure 2.6c shows an arterial phase CT image with a small hypervascular lesion in segment 2 of the left lobe of the liver and a tiny hypervascular lesion anteriorly in segment 4a of the right lobe.
- Figure 2.6d shows two similar lesions in segment 7 and one in segment 5/6.
- The appearance is in keeping with hypervascular liver metastases.

Principal diagnosis

- Small bowel carcinoid with liver metastases resulting in carcinoid syndrome.

Differential diagnosis

- Metastatic spread to the small bowel and liver or a primary small bowel carcinoma with liver metastases are possible but unlikely given the history of flushing and diarrhoea.

Table 2.6a Differential diagnosis

Causes of a desmoplastic reaction in the mesentery	Primary sites of tumours associated with hypervascular liver metastases
• Carcinoid	• Carcinoid
• Small bowel metastases	• Colon
	• Breast
	• Melanoma
	• Pancreatic islet cell tumour
	• Ovarian cystadenoma
• Lymphoma	• Sarcoma
• Fibrosing mesenteritis	• Phaeochromocytoma
• Desmoid tumour (FAP)	• Renal
	• Choriocarcinoma

(handwritten annotations: gastric, colon, breast cancer; pre-malignant lymphoma; orbital pseudotumour; thyroiditis; sclerosing cholangitis)

Further management

- ^{111}In-octreotide scan.
- MRI liver to assess the extent of the metastases.
- Referral to neuroendocrine cancer MDT for surgical resection of the primary tumour and treatment of the liver metastases.

Key points

- Gastrointestinal (GI) carcinoid is a malignant neuroendocrine tumor that arises within the enterochromaffin cells of Kulchitsky in the small bowel.
- 85% of all carcinoids arise in the GI tract.
- Rule of thirds:
  - one-third occur in the small bowel
  - one-third have metastases
  - one-third are multiple
  - one-third have a second malignancy.

- Occurs in the fifth to sixth decades.
- M:F = 2:1.
- On barium studies the lesions can present as submucosal filling defects, ulcerated target lesions, thickened mucosal folds, mesenteric retraction/tethering, and bowel dilatation.
- The classic appearance on CT is a mesenteric soft tissue mass with a 'spoke-wheel' desmoplastic reaction. Calcification is seen in up to 70%.
- Dilated thick-walled loops of small bowel due to bowel ischaemia are seen on CT and small bowel studies.
- GI carcinoids will be positive on ^{111}In-octreotide scan, ^{131}I-MIBG scan or somatostatin scintigraphy.
- Metastatic spread occurs to liver, lymph nodes, lung, and bone. Bone metastases are typically sclerotic.
- Liver metastases are usually hyperdense on the arterial phase.
- Carcinoid syndrome is caused by excess serotonin levels and requires that serotonin metabolism in the liver is bypassed. This occurs with metastatic spread to the liver or carcinoid outside the GI tract such as pulmonary or ovarian carcinoid. Symptoms included cutaneous flushing, wheezing, and diarrhoea.
- Treatment is with surgical excision of the primary bowel tumour and involved mesentery. Liver metastases can be treated by resection, chemoembolization, or radiofrequency ablation.
- The somatostatin analogue octreotide can be given for symptomatic relief.
- The 5 year survival rate for small bowel carcinoid is 90%, reducing to 50% in the presence of liver metastases.

References

Dähnert W. *Radiology Review Manual* (6th edn). Lippincott–Williams & Wilkins, 2007

Federle M, Jeffrey RB, Anne VS. *Diagnostic Imaging: Abdominal*. Amirsys, 2004

Scarsbrook AF, Ganeshan A, Statham J. Anatomic and functional imaging of metastatic carcinoid tumors. *Radiographics* **27**: 455–77, 2007

Notes

Sclerotic bone metr

A

Bronchu

Bladder

Bowel

Carcinoid

Prostate , phaeochromocytoma

Melanoma

Lymphoma.

Exam 3

Case 3.1

Clinical details

A 35-year-old female patient with a short history of progressive shortness of breath and dry cough.

Imaging

Figure 3.1a Chest radiograph.
Figures 3.1b–e Axial HRCT chest, supine images.

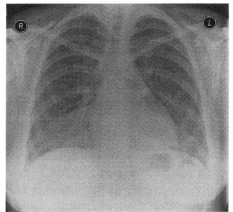

3.1a

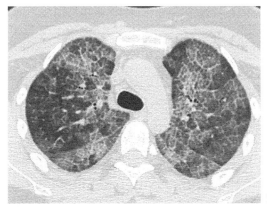

3.1b

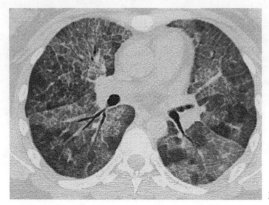

3.1c

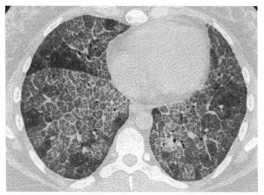

3.1d

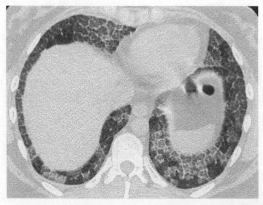

3.1e

Observations and interpretations

- Figure 3.1a shows diffuse bilateral alveolar shadowing. No pleural effusions. No cardiac enlargement.
- Figures 3.1b–e show a geographical 'crazy-paving' pattern of alveolar ground glass change with smooth septal thickening. The distribution of these changes is widespread with some sparing of the extreme periphery. There is clear demarcation between involved and uninvolved secondary pulmonary lobules (geographical sparing). No cardiac enlargement or pleural effusions. Normal airways. The main pulmonary artery is at the upper limit of normal for size.

Principal diagnosis

- Pulmonary alveolar proteinosis.

Differential diagnosis

- Pulmonary oedema.
- Pneumonia (especially *Pneumocystis carinii* pneumonia)
- Bronchoalveolar cell carcinoma.
- Alveolar haemorrhage.
- Adult respiratory distress syndrome (ARDS) (diffuse alveolar damage).
- Lymphangitis carcinomatosis.
- Hypersensitivity pneumonitis.
- Radiation damage.

[Handwritten margin notes:]
DDx crazy paving
unwell/immuno compromised
- PCP
- LVF
- RDS
- alveolar
well
- pulmonary haemorrhage
- lipoid pneumonia
- BAC

Table 3.1a Differential diagnosis of perihilar air-space shadowing on the chest radiograph

• Pulmonary oedema	• Perihilar air space shadowing: 'bat's wing' pattern • Kerley B lines of interstitial pulmonary oedema • Lamellar effusions (fluid between visceral pleura and lung) • Pleural effusions • Cardiomegaly (except in some cases of pulmonary oedema secondary to acute myocardial infarction) • Clinical symptoms usually severe and of sudden onset

• Pulmonary alveolar proteinosis	• Non-specific
	• Perihilar shadows:
	  • ground glass
	  • reticulonodular opacification
	  • consolidation
	• Sparing of the extremities on the chest radiograph
	• Absence of pleural effusions; the presence of effusions strongly suggests infection.
	• Heart size normal
	• Clinical symptoms moderate despite florid radiological abnormalities

• *Pneumocystis carinii* pneumonia	• Perihilar ground-glass and alveolar shadowing • Absence of lymphadenopathy and effusions • Pneumatocoele formation (especially upper zones)

Further management

- Bronchoalveolar lavage—this provides treatment and the diagnosis.

Key points   Nocardia infection.

- The pathology in alveolar proteinosis is due to a deficiency of pulmonary surfactant and impaired pulmonary immune function. This produces an abundance of lipoproteinaceous material which accumulates in the alveoli. It stains positively with periodic acid–Schiff (PAS).
- There are three groups of pulmonary alveolar proteinoses.
  - Idiopathic (90%)—high levels of antibodies against granulocyte–macrophage colony-stimulating factor (GM-CSF) in the blood and alveoli. This impairs surfactant and reduces antibacterial action.
  - Secondary to inhalation of inorganic dusts, haematological disorders, immune deficiency states (8%).
  - Congenital (2%)—severe hypoxaemia during the neonatal period (rare).
- Clinical—M:F = 3:1 in smokers, equal in non-smokers:
  - moderate symptoms—progressive dyspnoea and dry cough.
  - less commonly—fatigue, fever, weight loss.
- Increased incidence in smokers.
- HRCT—'crazy-paving' comprises smooth thickening of the septal lines and ground glass alveolar opacification. Interstitial oedema and engorged lymphatics are responsible for the septal thickening. There are various patterns ranging from focal and asymmetrical to diffuse and symmetrical. The area of affected lung correlates with physiological impairment. There is usually no air trapping.
- Treatment
  - Secondary—removal of agent responsible for lung changes.
  - Idiopathic—whole-lung bronchoalveolar lavage. This has improved prognosis and there is now a 95% survival rate following its introduction.
- Complications—secondary infection, respiratory failure.
- Other causes of mosaic attenuation
  - Air trapping in obliterative bronchiolitis (OB) and hypersensitivity pneumonitis (HP). The difference in attenuation between the affected and unaffected lung is exacerbated by expiratory views. The low-attenuation lung remains low density, whilst the higher-attenuation lung becomes denser during exhalation. This is because the small airways 'collapse' during exhalation since there is fibrosis (OB) or granulomata (HP) within the small airway walls. Pulmonary arteries are smaller in secondary pulmonary lobules that are less dense because of vasoconstriction associated with air trapping.
  - Vascular disease—pulmonary thromboembolic disease. Expiratory views should not cause air trapping in pure vascular disease. Obstruction to flow in pulmonary arteries causes a reduction in the size of the artery and low attenuation. This normalizes during exhalation as there is no associated airways disease.
  - Note that there may be combined vascular and small airways disease. Exhalation views can be employed to determine the dominant physiological effect.

Reference

Frazier AA, Franks TJ, Cooke EO, Mohammed TL, Pugatch RD, Galvin JR. From the archives of the AFIP: pulmonary alveolar proteinosis. *Radiographics* **28**: 883–99, 2008

Notes

Case 3.2

Clinical details

A 53-year-old male with raised calcium and hypertension.

Imaging

Figure 3.2a Thyroid ultrasound.

Figure 3.2b Thyroid ultrasound with colour Doppler (see also Plate 1).

Figure 3.2c Technetium-labelled sestamibi scan: planar images at 5min and 20min.

Figure 3.2d Technetium-labelled sestamibi scan: planar image at 2 hours.

Figure 3.2e Technetium-labelled sestamibi scan: SPECT image at 2 hours (see also Plate 2).

Figure 3.2f Axial short T1 inversion recovery (STIR) MRI of adrenals, unenhanced.

Figure 3.2g ^{123}I-MIBG whole-body scan.

Figure 3.2h ^{123}I-MIBG SPECT of abdomen (see also Plate 3).

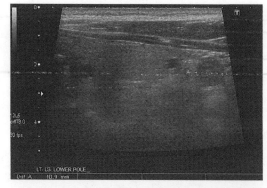

3.2a

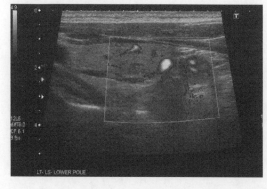

3.2b

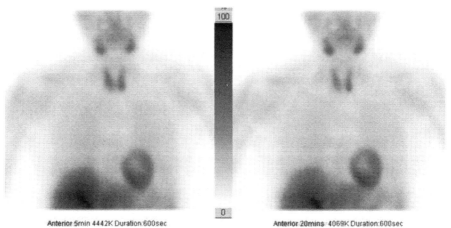

Anterior 5min 4442K Duration:600sec

Anterior 20mins 4069K Duration:600sec

3.2c

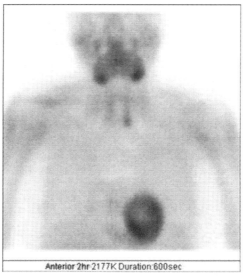

Anterior 2hr 2177K Duration:600sec

3.2d

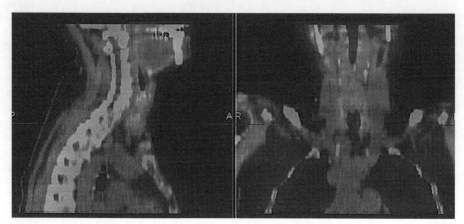

3.2e

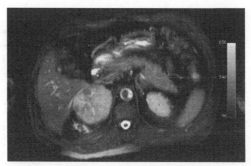

3.2f

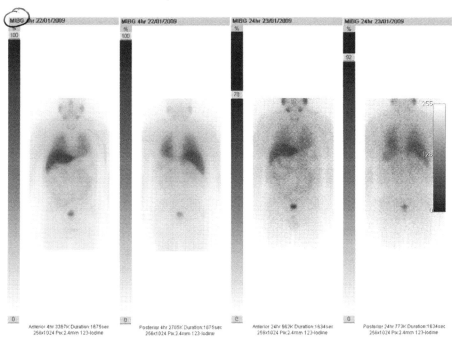

3.2g

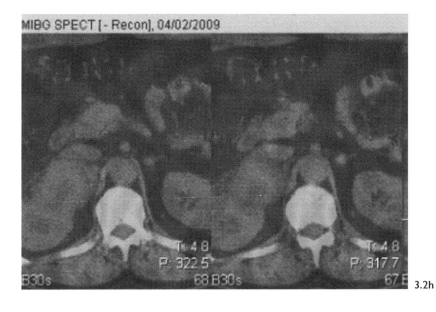

3.2h

Observations and interpretations

- Figures 3.2a and 3.2b show an 11mm rounded hypo-echoic lesion situated inferior to the left lobe of the thyroid. The lesion is hyper vascular on colour Doppler imaging.
- Figure 3.2c shows that there is physiological tracer activity in the salivary glands and in the thyroid gland, with a more prominent tracer focus in the region of the left thyroid lobe inferiorly. Figure 3.2d (delayed planar image at 2 hours) shows retention of this focus. Figure 3.2e (delayed SPECT image) localizes it inferior to the lower pole of the left thyroid lobe. This also correlates with the abnormality shown on ultrasound. The findings are in keeping with a left-sided parathyroid adenoma.
- Figure 3.2f shows a large right adrenal mass with mixed signal intensity. The differential diagnosis for this is a phaeochromocytoma, an adrenal carcinoma, or a metastasis.
- Figures 3.2g and 3.2h show physiological tracer activity in the liver. There is no abnormal tracer activity in the right adrenal mass which makes this less likely to be a phaeochromocytoma and more likely to be an adrenal carcinoma.

Principal diagnosis

- Multiple endocrine neoplasia syndrome type 1 (MEN-1) consisting of a left inferior pole parathyroid adenoma and a right adrenal carcinoma.

Differential diagnosis

- MEN-2 is associated with parathyroid adenomas and phaeochromocytomas. However, the lack of activity in the right adrenal mass on the MIBG scan makes diagnosis of a phaeochromocytoma unlikely.

Table 3.2a Differential diagnosis

Neck mass below thyroid gland	Adrenal mass
• Parathyroid adenoma	• Adrenal carcinoma
	• Phaeochromocytoma
• Thyroid nodule	• Metastastasis
• Lymph node	• Adrenal adenoma
	• Adrenal myelolipoma
	• Lymphoma
	• Neuroblastoma (child)
	• Haemorrhage

Further management

- Correlation with serum calcium and parathormone levels, urinary metanephrine, and catecholamines.
- Serum calcitonin levels and thyroid ultrasound to exclude medullary thyroid carcinoma.
- Surgical referral for the left parathyroid adenoma.
- Staging and surgical referral for the right adrenal carcinoma.
- Family history and genetic referral.

Key points

- MEN-1 is also known as Wermer's syndrome.
- Autosomal dominant condition with a high penetrance.
- M:F = 1:1.

- Genetic defect on chromosome 11.
- Features of MEN-1: (P x 3)
  - parathyroid adenoma/ hyperplasia (95%)
  - pancreatic islet cell tumour (40%)
  - anterior pituitary tumour (30%).
- Associated tumours:
  - facial angiofibroma (85–90%)
  - collagenoma (70%)
  - adrenal cortical tumour—adenomas and carcinomas (40%)
  - lipoma (10–30%)
  - foregut carcinoid (3–4%).

imaging surveillance:
renal u/s + AXR for calculi
Abdo MR for pancreal, adrenal
+ liver met.
pituitary MR for adenoma
every 3 years.

References

Carney JA. Familial multiple endocrine neoplasia syndromes: components, classification and nomenclature. *Journal of Internal Medicine* 243: 425–32, 1998

Marx SJ, Stratakis CA. Multiple endocrine neoplasia. *Journal of Internal Medicine* 257: 2–5, 2005.

Scarsbrook AF, Thakker RV, Wass JAH, Gleeson FV, Phillips RR. Multiple endocrine neoplasia: spectrum of radiologic appearances and discussion of a multitechnique imaging approach. *Radiographics* 26: 433–51, 2006.

Turner HE, Wass JAH. Multiple endocrine neoplasia. In: Turner HE (ed.) *Oxford Handbook of Endocrinology and Diabetes.* Oxford University Press, 2002; 718–30.

Notes

MEN type 2A   PPT
- parathyroid adenoma
- phaechromocytoma
- medullary thyroid carcinoma
* Surveillance
  ↳ abdominal MR every 3 years for phaechromocytoma.

MEN type 2B   PIM
- medullary thyroid carcinoma
- phaechromocytoma
- intestinal ganglioneuromatosis

Case 3.3

Clinical details

A 15-month-old baby presenting with recurrent episodes of crying and drawing up of the legs.

Imaging

Figure 3.3a Control fluoroscopic image taken with the patient in the prone position.
Figure 3.3b Ultrasound image of the upper abdomen.
Figure 3.3c Ultrasound image of the upper abdomen with colour Doppler imaging (see also Plate 4).

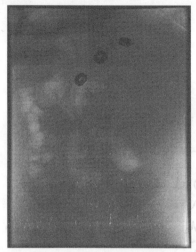

3.3a

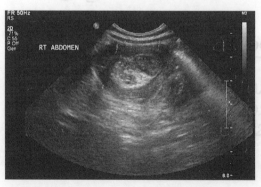

3.3b

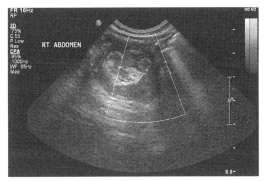

3.3c

Observations and interpretations

- Figure 3.3a shows a lack of gas in the right side of the abdomen. There is the impression of a soft tissue filling defect in the mid transverse colon. The descending colon is collapsed, and there are one or two dilated central small bowel loops. No free air is demonstrated.
- Figures 3.3b and c show a soft tissue mass with a 'target' or 'bull's eye' appearance, in keeping with an intussusception. The peripheral hypo-echoic ring represents the wall of the intussuscipiens, the central hyper-echoic area represents the mesenteric fat, and the internal hypo-echoic area is the intussuceptum. There is central vascularity with Doppler colour flow imaging. No fluid is demonstrated.

Principal diagnosis

- Idiopathic ileocolic intussusception.

Differential diagnosis

- None in this case.

Further management

- Reduction using air or gastrografin in the absence of any contraindications such as peritonitis, perforation, or shock.

Key points

- Intussusception is the most common cause of small bowel obstruction in childhood.
- The peak age is between 6 months and 2 years.
- M:F = 2:1.
- Clinical presentation is with a sudden onset of abdominal cramps, vomiting, and the passage of bloody or 'red currant jelly' stools.
- Over 95% of cases in childhood are idiopathic and are due to mucosal oedema and lymphoid hyperplasia of mucosa secondary to a viral gastroenteritis. The most common site for this is at the ileocaecal valve.
- In 5% of cases an underlying lead point is established. These include Meckel's diverticulum (most common), polyps, duplication cysts, tumours, appendicitis, and Henoch–Schönlein purpura.
- Typically ileocolic intussusception occurs more frequently than ileo-ileal intussusception. Colo-colic intussusception is the least frequent type.
- The intussusceptum (the internal loop of proximal bowel) prolapses into the intussuscipiens (the external loop of distal bowel). Vascular compromise of the mesenteric vessels may occur, resulting in bowel infarction.
- Plain films may show a soft tissue mass and small bowel obstruction. However, they may be normal in 25% of cases. comment on 'no free intrapen bowel air,,
- Transverse ultrasound scanning shows the typical 'target' or 'bull's eye sign', representing concentric rings of alternating hypo- and hyper-echoic layers of bowel wall.
- Longitudinal ultrasound scanning shows the 'pseudo-kidney sign'.
- Poor prognostic sonographic features include free intraperitoneal fluid, absent blood flow within the intussusception on colour Doppler imaging, and fluid between the intussusceptum and the intussuscipiens.
- CT also demonstrates a target appearance due to the layers of the intussusceptum/intussuscipiens and central low attenuation mesenteric fat.

- Reduction can be performed using air or gastrografin–water. However, it is <u>contraindicated</u> in the presence of <u>peritonitis</u>, <u>perforation</u>, or <u>shock</u>.
- The <u>intussusceptum is pushed back along the ascending colon until air fills small bowel, indicating</u> <u>a successful reduction</u>.

References

Dähnert W. *Radiology Review Manual* (6th edn). Lippincott–Williams & Wilkins, 2007

Daneman A, Navarro O. Intussusception. Part 1: A review of diagnostic approaches. *Pediatric Radiology* **33**: 79–85, 2003

del Pozo G, Albillos JC, Tejedor D, et al. Intussusception in children: current concepts in diagnosis and enema reduction. *Radiographics* **19**: 299–319, 1999

Hryhorczuk AL, Strouse PJ. Validation of US as a first-line diagnostic test for assessment of pediatric ileocolic intussusception. *Pediatric Radiology* **39**: 1075–9, 2009

Notes

mo-
yearr

Intussusception ⟵ Primary
          Secondary ⟹ leading point (si.)

└ hyper
   ┌ ileo-colic (most common)
   ├ ileo-ileal
   └ colo-colonic

   ┌ Meckel's (most common)
   ├ polyps
   ├ duplication cyst
   ├ tumour
   ├ appendicitis
   └ purpura Henoch-Schonlein

uls signs — "target" or "bull's eye sign"
            — "pseudokidney"

Poor prognostic signs ┌ free fluid
                      ├ absent flow
                      └ fluid between intussusceptum and intussuscipiens

Contraindication to air reduction
   ┌ peritonitis
   ├ shock
   └ perforation

Case 3.4

Clinical details

A 55-year-old male patient presenting with lethargy and back pain.

Imaging

Figure 3.4a Coronal CT image of the abdomen.
Figure 3.4b Sagittal CT image of the spine.
Figure 3.4c Sagittal T2W MRI of the spine.
Figure 3.4d Sagittal T1W MRI of the spine.

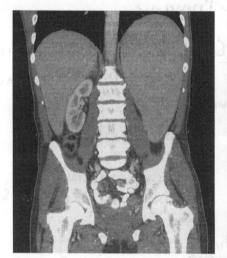
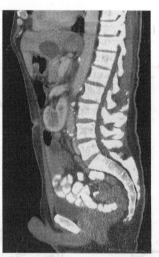

3.4a   3.4b

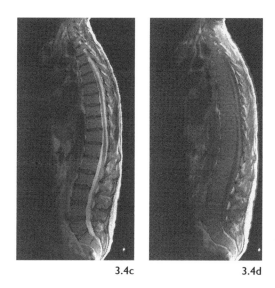

3.4c   3.4d

Observations and interpretations

- Figure 3.4a shows massive splenomegaly. No obvious abnormality is shown in the liver or remainder of the upper abdomen. No pathological lymph nodes demonstrated.
- Figure 3.4b shows diffuse osteosclerosis in the vertebral bodies. No evidence of vertebral body collapse. No bone destruction. The disc spaces are well maintained.
- Figures 3.4c and 3.4d show diffuse low-signal change within the bone marrow of the visualized vertebral bodies on the T1W and T2W images. On the T1W images the intervertebral discs are brighter than the bone marrow, which is the reverse of normal. No abnormality shown in the spinal cord or intervertebral discs.
- The appearances are those of either diffuse bone marrow infiltration or replacement.

Principal diagnosis

- Myelofibrosis

Differential diagnosis

- Lymphoma
- Leukaemia
- The above are less likely because of the presence of diffuse sclerosis.

Table 3.4a Differential diagnosis

Causes of diffuse low-signal change in the bone marrow on T1W and T2W images	Causes of diffuse osteosclerosis	Causes of massive splenomegaly
• **Myelofibrosis** • Chronic myeloid leukaemia • Lymphoma • Gaucher's disease • Metastases • Multiple myeloma • Haemosiderosis • Thalassaemia • Sickle cell anaemia	• **Myelofibrosis** • Metastases • Mastocytosis • Osteopetrosis • Fluorosis • Renal osteodystophy	• **Myelofibrosis** • Chronic myeloid leukaemia • Lymphoma • Gaucher's disease • Malaria • Kala azar

Further management

- Haematological referral/bone marrow biopsy.
- No further radiological management.

Key points

- The primary form of myelofibrosis may be a precursor to polycythaemia vera and chronic myeloid leukaemia. More commonly it is a secondary phenomenon due to leukaemia, lymphoma, or metastatic tumour.
- Myelofibrosis is characterized by the abnormal maturation of red blood cells and granulocytes and affects approximately 1 in 100,000 people. The median age at diagnosis is 60 years.
- Clinical presentation includes symptoms of fatigue, weight loss, easy bruising and bleeding, fever, night sweats, and hepatosplenomegaly.

- Gout and renal colic may occur due to hyperuricaemia from high cell turnover.
- The disease may be asymptomatic in up to 25% of patients.
- Bone marrow biopsy may be difficult and often reveals fibrosis with variable degrees of marrow hyperplasia.
- The radiographic hallmark of myelofibrosis is osteosclerosis, most commonly found in the axial skeleton and the proximal aspects of the long bones.
- Osteosclerosis is due to the replacement of the normal marrow cavity with fibrous tissue with no trabecular or cortical disorganization.
- The loss of the normal high-signal fatty marrow on T1W images and the decreased signal on T2W images is due to the marrow's abnormal hypercellularity.
- Myelofibrosis may be cured by allogenic bone marrow transplantation. Other forms of therapy are palliative and are used primarily to improve anaemia (androgens with or without steroids, thalidomide, splenectomy, splenic radiation), to reduce symptoms related to organomegaly and hypermetabolism (chemotherapy), or to treat complications (allopurinol for treatment of hyperuricaemia).
- Causes of death are variable in myelofibrosis and include leukaemic conversion in 5–20% and overwhelming infection, haemorrhage, cardiovascular events, thrombosis, renal failure, and hepatic failure.
- The most common difficulty in bone marrow interpretation is distinguishing neoplastic marrow infiltration from red bone marrow reconversion.
- At birth, the skeleton is composed of haematopoietic red marrow that matures to yellow or fatty marrow with age. The process typically progresses from peripheral to central, although the rate and pattern of progression can vary. Red bone marrow reconversion refers to the process of mature yellow marrow being replaced by haematopoietic red marrow.
- Red marrow reconversion has many causes, including physiological stress, smoking, marrow-stimulating medications, and living at high altitude.
- On T1W images, red marrow has decreased signal compared with yellow marrow, but remains hyperintense to skeletal muscle. Neoplastic marrow infiltration is typically isointense or hypointense to skeletal muscle on T1W images.

References

Cloran F, Banks KP. AJR Teaching file: diffuse osteosclerosis with hepatosplenomegaly. *American Journal of Roentgenology* **188**: S18–20, 2007

Long SS, Yablon CM, Eisenberg RL. Bone Marrow marrow signal alteration in the spine and sacrum. *American Journal of Roentgenology* **195**: W178–200, 2010

Swartz PG, Roberts CC. Radiological reasoning: bone marrow changes on MRI. *American Journal of Roentgenology* **193**: S1–4, 2009

Notes

Case 3.5

Clinical details

A 50-year-old female patient with symptoms of sinusitis and haemoptysis.

Imaging

Figures 3.5a–b Coronal CT scans of the sinuses.
Figures 3.5c–d Axial CT scans of the lungs.

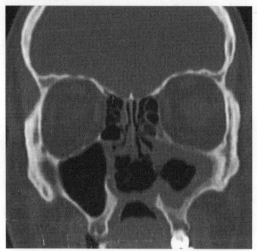

3.5a

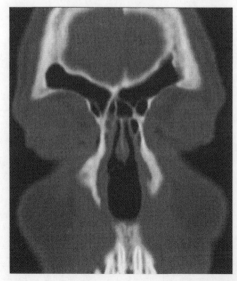

3.5b

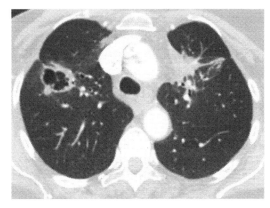

3.5c

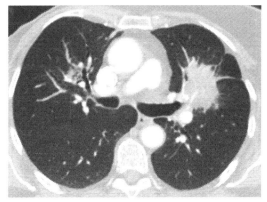

3.5d

Observations and interpretations

- Figures 3.5a and 3.5b show a destructive process involving the nose and paranasal sinuses. There is destruction of the hard palate, medial walls of both maxillary sinuses, nasal septum, and middle and inferior turbinates. There is a rind of soft tissue in the left maxillary sinus, along the medial wall of the right maxillary sinus and floor of the nasal passage.
- Figures 3.5c and 3.5d show a thick-walled cavity in the right upper lobe of the lung and a soft tissue mass in the left upper lobe adjacent to the left hilum. There is some pleural retraction in the lateral aspect of the chest. No lymphadenopathy, collapse, or effusions are shown on the images.

Principal diagnosis

- Wegener's granulomatosis.

Differential diagnosis

- Invasive fungal sinusitis and fungal infection in the lungs—unlikely unless the patient was immunocompromised.

Table 3.5a Differential diagnosis

Causes of a destructive midline sinonasal process	Causes of thick-walled cavitating lung lesions
• Wegener's granulomatosis • Invasive fungal sinusitis • T-cell lymphoma • Cocaine abuse	• Wegener's granulomatosis • Infections: fungal (aspergillus, cryptococcus), mycobacterial (tuberculosis), bacterial (gram-negative, *Staphylococcus aureus*), parasitic (echinococcus) • Metastases: squamous cell carcinoma, sarcoma, colon, melanoma, transitional cell carcinoma, cervix, post chemotherapy, seminoma, Wilms' tumour • Septic emboli, pulmonary embolus with infarction • Rheumatoid, systemic lupus erythematosus

Further management

- ENT referral and biopsy of soft tissue in nasal passage.
- Chest referral and consider CT-guided lung biopsy if the diagnosis was not established by nasal biopsy.
- Correlation with renal function and classical antineutrophil cytoplasmic antibody (c-ANCA).

Key points

- Wegener's granulomatosis is a necrotizing granulomatous vasculitis of small to medium-sized vessels.
- Mean age at diagnosis is 40–55 years.
- M:F = 1:1. More common in Caucasians.
- Wegener's granulomatosis can affect any part of the body. However, it typically presents with involvement of the sinuses, lungs, and kidneys.
- The clinical presentation is wide ranging with signs and symptoms of sinusitis, cough, fever, haemoptysis, proteinuria, and haematuria.

Triad ← respiratory tract inflammation.
       ← small vessel vasculitis.
       ← necrotizing glomerulonephritis,

- Pulmonary involvement includes multiple cavitating lung nodules which tend to be adjacent to bronchi or subpleural in location. The nodules range in size up to 10cm and can have ill-defined margins or a halo sign due to surrounding haemorrhage. Cavitation is seen in 50% — the cavities can be thick or thin-walled. Rapid enlargement may be due to haemorrhage or infection. The nodules can regress spontaneously. Stenosis of the peripheral airways may result in segmental atelectasis. Confluent areas of consolidation may occur due to haemorrhage.
- Tracheal stenosis is also associated and occurs later in the disease. The most common site is in the subglottic area. (ΔΔx relapsing polychondritis →nosincer disease)
- Pleural effusions are seen in 20%. Pneumothoraces and mediastinal lymphadenopathy are rare.
- Lung changes start to clear one week post-treatment and usually resolve by one month.
- Renal failure secondary to focal necrotizing glomerulonephritis is the most common cause of death.
- Sinus changes include nasal septal perforation, lateral nasal wall destruction, and paranasal sinus inflammatory change. Septal perforation leads to saddle-nose deformity.
- The diagnosis is made by renal, sinus, or lung biopsy. 70–90% of patients with Wegener's granulomatosis have a positive c-ANCA test which supports the diagnosis. However, this is not necessary to make the diagnosis.
- Treatment is with steroids and cyclophosphamide. There is an increased risk of myeloproliferative disorder and transitional cell carcinoma with cyclophosphamide therapy.
- Tracheobronchial stenosis can be treated with stent placement.
- Survival at 24 months is 80%; relapse occurs in 50% and drug toxicity in 42%.

References

Stern M, Winer-Muram H. *Diagnostic Imaging: Chest.* Amirsys, 2006
Harnsberger HR. *Pocket Radiologist: Head and Neck. Top 100 Diagnoses.* Amirsys, 2002

Notes

Lung cavities.
- Infection ← Bacterial ← st. aureus / klebsiella
                ← TB
                ← fungal: aspergillosis
- Malignancy ← Bronchus - squamous cell
                ← Met - scc, colon, sarcoma.
                ← Hodgkin's
- Infarction - PE
- inflammatory / Granloma ← wegener's
                ← RA
                ← SLE
                ← PMF
                ← sarcoid.
- Traumatic ← haematoma
             ← traumatic lung cyst
- Septic emboli
- Abnormal lung ← infective emphysematous bulla.
                ← Sequestrated segment
                ← Bronchogenic cyst.

Case 3.6

Clinical details

A 28-year-old women referred to the regional liver unit following a routine ultrasound scan for the exclusion of gallstones.

Imaging

Figure 3.6a Sagittal ultrasound image of the left lobe of the liver pre (left hand image) and post IV contrast (right hand image) (see also Plate 5).

Figure 3.6b T1W MRI through the upper abdomen.

Figure 3.6c Fat-suppressed T2W MRI through the upper abdomen.

Figure 3.6d Dynamic fat-suppressed T1W post-gadolinium image in the arterial phase.

Figure 3.6e Dynamic fat-suppressed T1W post-gadolinium image in the portal venous phase.

Figure 3.6f Dynamic fat-suppressed T1W post-gadolinium image in the delayed phase.

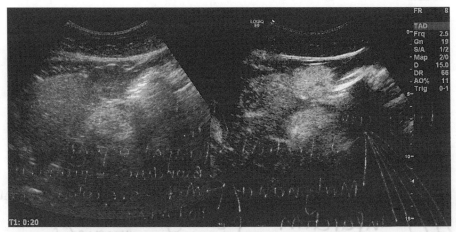

3.6a

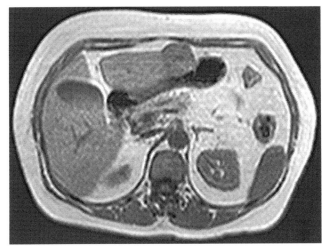

3.6b

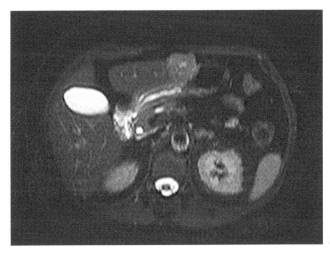

3.6c

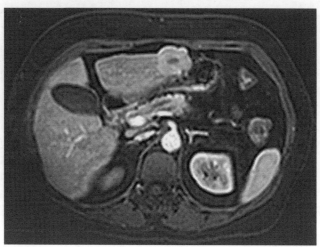

3.6d

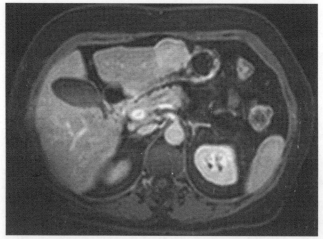

3.6e

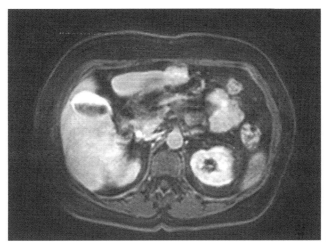

3.6f

Observations and interpretations

- Figure 3.6a shows a focal lesion in the liver with uniform uptake of microbubbles.
- Figures 3.6b and 3.6c show a 4cm hypoechoic lesion in the left lobe of the liver which is slightly hypo-intense to normal liver on T1W and hyper-intense to normal liver on the fat-suppressed T2W image.
- There is evidence of a central scar which is of low signal intensity on T1W and high signal intensity on T2W.
- Figure 3.6d shows evidence of peripheral enhancement on the arterial phase with a low-signal central scar. Figure 3.6e shows that the lesion enhances uniformly on the portal venous phase, and Figure 3.6f shows that there is uptake within the central scar on the delayed phase.
- Several gallstones are also noted in the gall bladder.

Principal diagnosis

- Focal nodular hyperplasia.

Differential diagnosis

- Hepatic adenoma—less likely. A central scar is not typical of an adenoma.
- Fibrolamellar carcinoma—unlikely in view of the patient's age. There are no features of malignancy such as local invasion or nodal metastases.

Further management

- Discussion at the hepatobiliary multidisciplinary meeting.
- Discontinue the oral contraceptive pill if necessary.
- Usually no further treatment is needed as it is rarely symptomatic.

Key points

- Focal nodular hyperplasia is thought to occur because of a proliferation of hepatocytes secondary to a vascular malformation.
- Asymptomatic in up to 90% of cases.
- Typically found in females in the third and fourth decades.
- Rarely needs treatment except for cessation of the pill because of its effect on growth.
- 20% are classified as atypical. They may show features of adenomas but all lack the classical features as described. These tumours require follow-up with serial scanning. Hepatocyte-specific contrast agents may be helpful.
- Hepatic adenoma. May be symptomatic secondary to haemorrhage. Associated with the oral contraceptive pill. May increase in size in pregnancy. Usually heterogeneous on imaging because of haemorrhage, necrosis, or fat.
- Fibrolamellar carcinoma. Usually large mass (more than 12cm) which is more heterogeneous in signal intensity. The scar is usually of low signal intensity on T2W. Associated findings are invasion of bile ducts and vessels. Nodal/distant metastatic disease is seen in 70%.

References

Anderson SW, Kruskal JB, Kane RA. Benign hepatic tumors and iatrogenic pseudotumors. *Radiographics* **29**: 211–29, 2009

Silva AC, Evans JM, McCullough AE, Jatoi MA, Vargas HE, Hara AK. MR imaging of hyper-vascular liver masses: a review of current techniques. *Radiographics* **29**: 385–402, 2009

Gandhi SN, Brown MA, Wong JG, Aguirre DA, Sirlin CB. MR contrast agents for liver imaging: what, when, how. *Radiographics* **26**: 1621–36, 2006

Notes

Exam 4

Case 4.1

Clinical details

A 70-year-old male with wheeze, cough, and intermittent dyspnoea.

Imaging

Figure 4.1a Chest radiograph.
Figure 4.1b–c HRCT of the chest.
Figure 4.1d Chest radiograph, 3 years after presentation.
Figure 4.1e–f HRCT of the chest, 3 years after presentation.

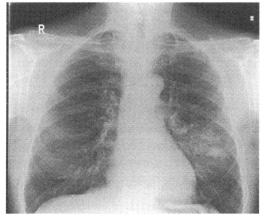

4.1a

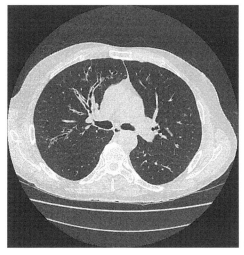

4.1b

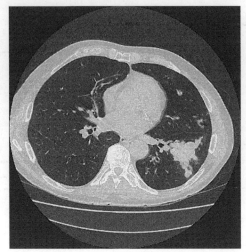

4.1c

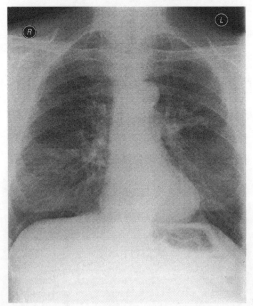

4.1d

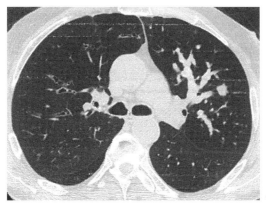

4.1e

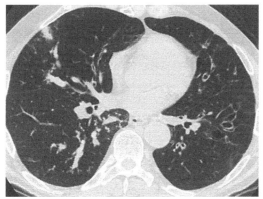

4.1f

Observations and interpretations

- Figure 4.1a demonstrates an infiltrate and a cluster of large-calibre tubular opacities in the left mid zone. There are small-calibre tubular opacities ('tramline opacities') in the right upper lobe. No pleural effusions or cardiac enlargement.
- Figures 4.1b and 4.1c show a cluster of tubular opacities in the left lower lobe, which has an appearance like 'gloved fingers' (bronchoceles) due to mucoid impaction. There is central cylindrical bronchiectasis in the right upper lobe.
- Figure 4.1d (3 years later) demonstrates bronchoceles in both mid-zones but in different locations. No pleural effusions or cardiac enlargement.
- Figures 4.1e and 4.1f (3 years later) show central bronchoceles with 'gloved fingers' appearance in the left upper lobe and right upper and lower lobes. Bronchiectasis without bronchoceles is seen in the left lower lobe. There are also small nodules in the right lower lobe, in keeping with a 'tree in bud' appearance indicating endobronchial infection.
- Central bronchiectasis and bronchoceles are demonstrated with changing locations over a 3 year interval.

Principal diagnosis

- Allergic bronchopulmonary aspergillosis (ABPA).

Differential diagnosis

- None

Further management

- Serological tests (see below)

Key points

- ABPA is a hypersensitivity reaction (types I and III) to *Aspergillus fumigatus* antigen and is typically seen in asthmatics or patients with cystic fibrosis.
- 10% of cystic fibrosis patients have ABPA.
- Early signs on chest radiograph—fleeting alveolar infiltrates (probable eosinophilic pneumonia) which tend to 'move around' the radiograph with time.
- Later signs—consolidation leads to damage to the bronchial wall with bronchiectasis and mucoid impaction. Chronic infiltrates may cavitate (20%).
- ABPA is diagnosed when the following are present:
  - asthma
  - peripheral eosinophilia (>1000/µl)
  - positive skin-prick test and antibodies to *Aspergillus fumigatus* antigen
  - raised serum IgE (and raised serum IgE and IgG to *Aspergillus fumigatus* antigen)
  - constant or fleeting pulmonary infiltrates on chest radiograph
  - central bronchiectasis (mainly involving upper lobes).
- Radiological findings highly suggestive of ABPA include:
  - bronchiectasis of three or more lobes
  - centrilobular nodules
  - mucoid impaction (high attenuation due to calcium deposition).
- Other findings include air trapping, collapse/atelectasis, and consolidation.

References

Buckingham SJ, Hansell DM. Aspergillus in the lung: diverse and coincident forms. *European Radiology* **13**: 1786–1800, 2003

Martinez S, Heyneman LE, McAdams HP, Rossi SE, Restrepo CS, Eraso A. Mucoid impactions: finger-in-glove sign and other CT and radiographic features. *Radiographics* **28**: 1369–82, 2008

Notes

Recurrent Fleeting Infiltrates

- simple pulmonary eosinophilia
- bronchopulmonary aspergillosis.
- asthma
- subacute bacterial endocarditis c̄ pulmonary emboli [± cavitation]
- pulmonary haemorrhage
- pulmonary vasculitis
- COP
- recurrent aspiration

Case 4.2

Clinical details

A 21-year-old female patient presenting with a 3-day history of headache and vomiting.

Imaging

Figure 4.2a Axial unenhanced CT of brain.
Figure 4.2b Axial gradient-recalled echo (GRE) MRI.
Figure 4.2c Sagittal T1W MRI.
Figure 4.2d Sagittal magnetic resonance venography (MRV) of the dural venous sinuses, unenhanced

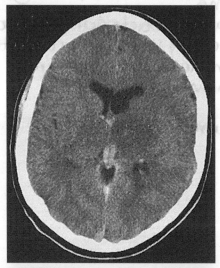

4.2a

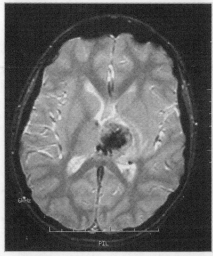

4.2b

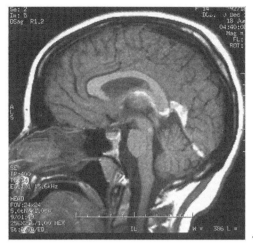

4.2c

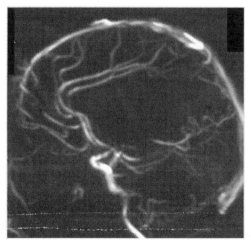

4.2d

Observations and interpretation

- Figure 4.2a shows a dense appearance of the straight sinus, in keeping with thrombus. In addition, there is a well-circumscribed area of low attenuation in the left thalamus with flecks of haemorrhage. There is a degree of mass effect with dilatation of the frontal horns of the lateral ventricles.
- Figure 4.2b shows low-signal change in the left thalamus, in keeping with haemosiderin from a recent haemorrhage. There is no significant surrounding cerebral oedema.
- Figure 4.2c shows high-signal filling defects in the straight sinus, the vein of Galen, and the basal vein (Rosenthal vein), in keeping with thrombus.
- Figure 4.2d demonstrates absence of flow in the inferior sagittal sinus and the straight sinus, and also in both the transverse sigmoid sinuses and the jugular veins.

internal cerebral a & vein

Principal diagnosis

- Thrombosis of the straight sinus/deep cerebral veins resulting in haemorrhagic infarct of the left thalamus.

Differential diagnosis

- None.

Further management

- Contrast-enhanced MRV of the dural venous sinuses to confirm extent of thrombosis.
- Specialist referral.
- Anticoagulant treatment.

Key points

- Uncommon condition—incidence 2–7 cases per million population.
- Clinical presentation—headache, seizures, focal neurological deficits.
- Non-contrast CT—thrombus appears as high-attenuation material in the sinus, most commonly affecting the superior sagittal and then the straight sinus.
- Contrast-enhanced CT—empty delta sign which represents central thrombus surrounded by contrast.

  isointense T1, MRV low signal T2 + Gd

- MRI—thrombus will have different signal intensities depending on the age. Acute thrombus has an intensity which may mimic normal flowing blood and therefore may be missed. Subacute thrombus appears high intensity on T1W and T2W imaging and therefore is easier to detect. Chronic thrombus may enhance due to intrinsic vascularization and therefore may also be difficult to detect.
- Focal brain abnormalities may be due to cytotoxic oedema, infarction, or haemorrhage.
- Post-contrast images may show areas of gyral enhancement as well as enhancement of the tentorium and meninges and prominent cortical venous enhancement.
- Haemorrhage occurs in a third of cases and typically occurs in a parasagittal location in superior sagittal sinus thrombosis. MRI with GRE sequences is most sensitive for detecting haemorrhage.
- Thalamic oedema is associated with thrombus in the straight sinus, the vein of Galen, or the internal cerebral veins. Deep venous occlusion presents with symptoms of raised intracranial pressure leading rapidly to coma.
- Local causes of dural venous sinus thrombosis:
  - tumour infiltrating sinus
  - trauma
  - regional infection (mastoiditis, empyema, abscess).

- Systemic causes of dural venous sinus thrombosis:
  - hypercoagulable states (pregnancy, oral contraceptive pill, septicaemia, malignancy, chemotherapy, idiopathic thrombocytosis, polycythaemia vera, sickle cell disease, etc.)
  - dehydration, shock, cardiac failure   ⊛ antiphospholipid syndrome ⊛
  - unknown cause in up to 25% of cases.

References

Greiner FG, Takhtani D. Neuroradiology case of the day. Superior sagittal sinus thrombosis. *Radiographics* **19**: 1098–1101, 1999

Leach JL, Fortuna RB, Jones BV, Gaskill-Shipley MF. Imaging of cerebral venous thrombosis: current techniques, spectrum of findings and diagnostic pitfalls. *Radiographics* **26**: S19–41, 2006

Notes

Superior cerebrum → Superior sagittal sinus
Peri-insular region → Sylvian veins
Temporal, parietal, occipital → transverse sinus
     └ vein of Labbé if prominent
Thalamus, caudate → vein of Galen (internal cerebral vein)

superior sagittal sinus

Troland

inferior sagittal

internal cerebral — straight

Thalamostriate (Thalamo mochriate) / vein of Galen — torcula / confluence
anterior thalamo
basal vein — cavernous — Labbé — transverse sinus
petrosal — sigmoid
jugular

- inferior frontal
- deep white matter
- temporal + parietal
- corpus callosum
     — basal ganglia — thalamus

Deep system
- vein of Galen
- internal cerebral
- rosenthal vein

Case 4.3

Clinical details

A 2-month-old boy presenting to A&E with failure to thrive.

Imaging

Figures 4.3a–c Chest X-ray and oblique views of the ribs.
Figure 4.3d X-ray of the lower limbs.
Figure 4.3e X-rays of the hands.
Figure 4.3f X-rays of the wrists.

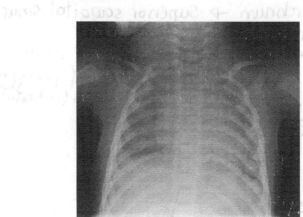

4.3a

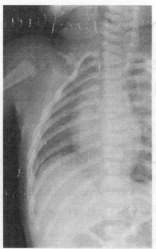

4.3b

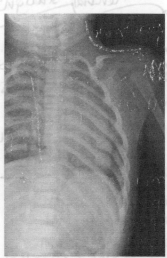

4.3c

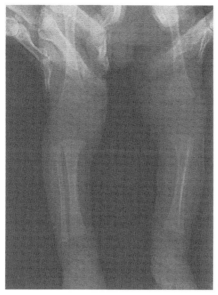

4.3d

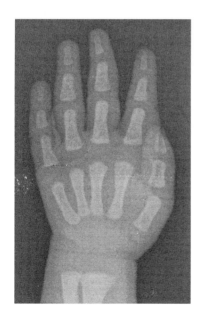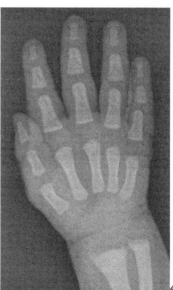

4.3e

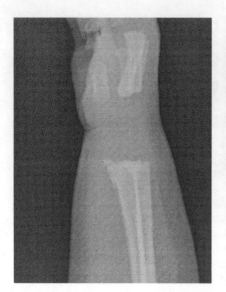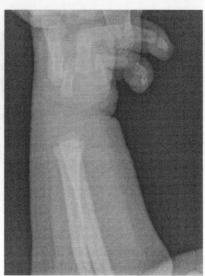

4.3f

Observations and interpretations

- Figures 4.3a–c show healing posterior rib fractures of the left fifth, sixth, seventh, and ninth ribs, and the right sixth and seventh ribs. There is also an old fracture of the right clavicle.
- Figure 4.3d shows a metaphyseal corner fracture at the medial aspect of the right distal femur and at the lateral aspect of the right distal fibula. There is a metaphyseal corner fracture at the medial aspect of the left distal femur with periosteal reaction along the femoral shaft.
- Figures 4.3e and 4.3f show a metaphyseal corner fracture of the right distal radius.

Principal diagnosis

- Non-accidental injury (NAI).

Differential diagnosis

- The presence of multiple asymmetrical fractures including posterior rib fractures and metaphyseal corner fractures is strongly suggestive of non accidental injury. Other diagnoses such as osteogenesis imperfecta, rickets and metaphyseal dysplasia are very unlikely.

Further management

- Concerns over suspected NAI should be raised immediately with the referring clinicians.
- A full radiographic skeletal survey ± cross-sectional imaging of the brain if there are any skull fractures or signs of head injury.

Key points

- Skeletal trauma occurs in 50–80% of NAI injury cases and is characterized by multiple fractures at different stages of repair.
- Metaphyseal, 'corner', or 'bucket-handle' fractures are avulsion injuries resulting from application of a sudden pulling or twisting force to the limb.
- Extensive periosteal reactions can occur as a result of subperiosteal haemorrhage.
- Posterior rib fractures typically occur as a result of application of a squeezing/crushing force to the chest.
- These fractures do not occur in normal infants as a result of normal handling and should always be accompanied by a clear account of the mechanism of injury.
- Osteogenesis imperfecta typically presents with long-bone shaft fractures associated with minor trauma. Other radiological features include Wormian bones and reduced bone density.
- Metaphyseal cupping, splaying, and fraying are typical features of rickets, but should be uniform and affect all metaphyses symmetrically. Rickets is not associated with rib fractures.
- Irregular metaphyses are seen in metaphyseal dysplasia, but the affected metaphyses are usually symmetrical and generalized. Metaphyseal dysplasias are not associated with rib fractures.
- A full radiographic skeletal survey consisting of 19 separate radiographs is recommended by the Royal College of Radiologists/Royal College of Paediatrics and Child Health (RCR/RCPH) when NAI is suspected.

References

Offiah A, van Rijn RR, Perez-Rossello JM, Kleinman PK. Skeletal imaging of child abuse (non-accidental injury). *Pediatric Radiology* **39**: 461–70

RCR/RCPH. *Standards of Imaging in Suspected Non-Accidental Injury*. RCR/RCPH, 2008

Notes

Standard skeletal survey

Skull — AP, lateral

Chest ⎡ AP (including clavicles)
⎣ oblique views both sides — ℝ, 𝕃.

Abdomen — AP.

Spine — lateral whole spine

Limbs ⎡ AP both upper arms
⎢ AP both upper fore-arms
⎢ PA both hands
⎢ AP both femur
⎢ AP both lower legs
⎣ DP both feet

* Followup CXR 4-6 weeks.

Indications neuro-imaging.

- age <1 → evident physical abuse.
= any age — physical abuse + encephalopathic
feature + focal neurology + retinopathy
+ abnormal neurology or encephalopathy

If CT HEAD Ⓝ → MRI day 3-5
⎡ T2 + TrWI
⎢ DWI → cytotoxic oedema → hypoxic
⎢ GRE ischaemic injury bilateral
⎣ → microhaemorrhage. changes

Case 4.4

Clinical details

A one-day-old infant presenting with persistent vomiting and abdominal distension.

Imaging

Figure 4.4a Plain abdominal X-ray.

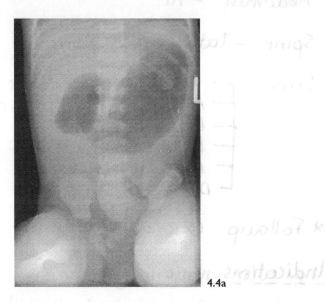

4.4a

Observations and interpretations

- There is gaseous distension of the stomach and the first part of the duodenum—'double-bubble sign'.
- There is no evidence of gas distally within the small or large bowel.
- No free air.

Principal diagnosis

- Duodenal atresia.

Differential diagnosis

- Duodenal web or duodenal stenosis may give a similar picture, but is usually associated with gas in the distal loops of bowel on the abdominal radiograph.
- External compression of the duodenum by a gastrointestinal (GI) duplication cyst or annular pancreas may also cause proximal dilatation of stomach and duodenum.

Further management

- Upper GI tract contrast study to confirm the diagnosis.
- Urgent referral to paediatric surgeons.
- Exclude other associated congenital anomalies such as Down's syndrome.

Key points

- Duodenal atrasia is the most common cause of congenital duodenal obstruction.
- Incidence 1:10,000; M:F = 1:1.
- Presents in the first few days of life with persistent vomiting and rapid dehydration due to fluid loss.
- Obstruction of the bowel, usually in the second or third part of the duodenum in the region of the ampulla of Vater.
- Occurs due to defective vacuolization of the duodenum in weeks 6–11 of life. Rarely occurs as the result of a vascular insult.
- Associated with Down's syndrome—25% of cases of duodenal atresia have trisomy 21.
- Other associated features include congenital heart disease (endocardial cushion defect, ventricular septal defect), GI tract abnormalities (malrotation, annular pancreas, oesophageal/biliary/small bowel atresia), urinary tract abnormalities, vertebral and rib abnormalities.
- The classic finding on plain film is the 'double-bubble sign' of an air–fluid level in the stomach and duodenum.
- There is a total absence of gas in the remaining small/large bowel.
- Can be diagnosed on obstetric ultrasound after 24 weeks. Associated with polyhydramnios and increased gastric peristalsis.
- Upper GI contrast study can be helpful to differentiate from other causes of obstruction.
- If there is proximal obstruction with gas in the distal loops, mid-gut volvulus must also be considered.
- Associated with preterm labour due to polyhydramnios.

References

Dähnert W. *Radiology Review Manual* (6th edn). Lippincott–Williams & Wilkins, 2007

Dalla Vecchia LK, Grosfeld JL, West KW, Rescorla FJ, Scherer LR, Engum SA. Intestinal atresia and
    stenosis: a 25-year experience with 277 cases. *Archives of Surgery* **133**: 490–7, 1998
Donnelly L (ed). *Diagnostic Imaging: Pediatrics.* Amirysys, 2005

Notes

Duodenal atresia ⟶ Proximal obstruction
  Duodenal stenosis
    Duodenal webs
      Annular pancreas
        Peritoneal Ladder
        Preduodenal portal vein
              Malrotation volvulus.

High intestinal obstruction
              jejunal atresia.

Low intestinal obstruction
              ileal
              jejunal atresia.
              meconium ileus
              colonic atresia.
              meconium plug syndrome.
              Hischprung's
              incarcerated inguinal hernia
              small left colon
              anorectal malformation/imperforate anus

Case 4.5

Clinical details:

A 24-year-old female brought into AED following horse riding accident. Patient had free fluid on FAST (focused assessment with sonography for trauma) scanning and proceeded to emergency laparotomy. Following stabilization the patient underwent CT scanning

Imaging

Figs 4.5a–d CT scan of upper abdomen post intravenous contrast

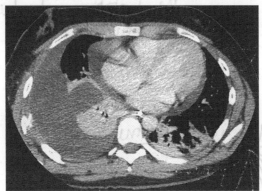

4.5a

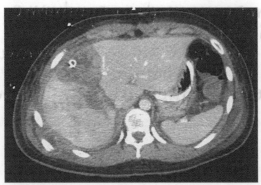

4.5b

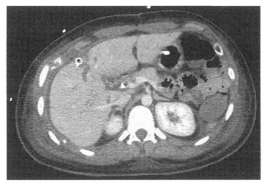

4.5c

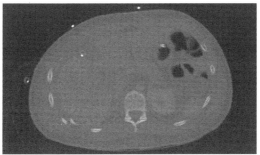

4.5d

Observations and interpretation

- Figure 4.5a shows a large right pleural effusion, pericardial effusion, bibasal lung atelectasis, and right-sided rib fractures.
- Figure 4.5b shows a nasogastric tube *in situ* and a right subphrenic drain. The liver is abnormal. There is a low attenuation area extending down through segments 7–8 towards the hilum of the liver. The appearances are in keeping with a liver laceration.
- There is a trace of free fluid around the liver and the spleen.
- The spleen is intact and perfused.
- Both kidneys excrete contrast.
- There is no intraperitoneal gas to suggest bowel laceration.
- Figure 4.5d shows the right rib fractures on bone window settings.

Principal diagnosis

- Liver laceration secondary to trauma with probable traumatic right pleural/pericardial effusions and right sided rib fractures.

Differential diagnosis

- None

Further management

- The patient if stable should be transferred to the regional liver unit for close observation.
- Serial CT as required to assess liver necrosis and possible sepsis advised.
- If the patient is unstable then assessment for haemorrhage or portosystemic fistula should be made with angiography.

Key points

- The liver is a frequently injured abdominal organ.
- Associated with splenic injury in 45%.
- Although FAST scanning is the most commonly used diagnostic imaging method in patients after major trauma, its role in the diagnosis of injuries to solid organs is limited. Reported values for the sensitivity of FAST in the detection of liver injuries range from 0.15 to 0.88.
- Multi-row detector CT is the imaging modality of choice. The typical appearance is a low-attenuation laceration which may be branching ± subcapsular haematoma. The liver may show wedge-shaped areas of devascularization. Hyperdense areas may suggest active haemorrhage or pseudo-aneurysm formation.
- Left lobe injuries may be associated with pancreas and root of mesentery injury. Always check abdomen on work station on lung windows to look for free air as well as on abdominal and liver settings.
- Treatment of choice is conservative with serial scanning ± angiography/embolization.
- The prognosis varies with the CT stage but other variables, such as other organ damage, need to be taken into account.

Table 4.5a Categories of liver injury on CT

Grade	Injury	Description
I	Haematoma	Subcapsular <10% of surface area
	Laceration	Capsular tear <1cm of parenchymal depth
II	Haematoma	Subcapsular 10–50% of surface area; intraparenchymal <10cm in diameter
	Laceration	1–3cm deep and <10cm long
III	Haematoma	Subcapsular >50% of surface area; ruptured subcapsular/parenchymal
	Laceration	Intraparenchymal >10cm/expanding; >3cm parenchymal depth
IV	Laceration	Parenchymal disruption 25–75% of lobe; 1–3 Couinaud segments in single lobe
V	Laceration	Disruption >75% of single lobe; >3 Couinaud segments in single lobe
	Vascular	Juxtahepatic venous injury (HV,IVC)
VI	Vascular	Hepatic avulsion

References

Becker CD, Gal I, Baer HU, Vock P. Blunt hepatic trauma in adults: correlation of CT injury grading with outcome. *Radiology* **201**: 215–20, 1996

Patten RM, Gunberg SR, Brandenburger DK, Richardson ML. CT detection of hepatic and splenic injuries: usefulness of liver window settings. *American Journal of Roentgenology* **175**: 1107–10, 2000

Tkacz JN, Anderson SA, Soto J. MR imaging in gastrointestinal emergencies. *Radiographics* **29**: 1767–80, 2009

Notes

Case 4.6

Clinical details

A 61-year-old female patient presenting with haematemesis.

Imaging

Figures 4.6a–c Selected axial CT images through the abdomen and pelvis.
Figures 39d–f Selected axial, sagittal, and coronal CT images through the upper abdomen 10 months later.

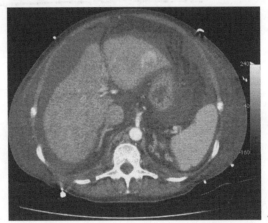

4.6a

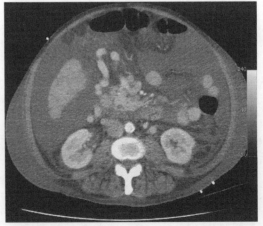

4.6b

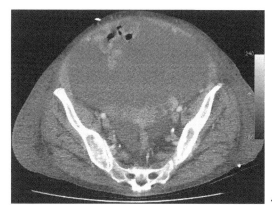

4.6c

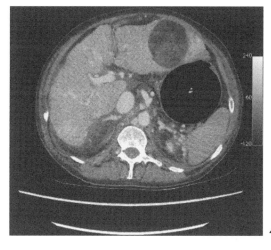

4.6d

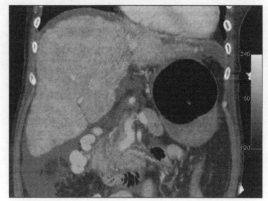

4.6e

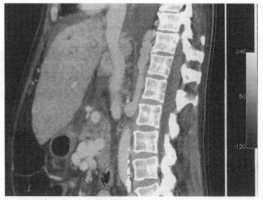

4.6f

Observations and interpretations

- Figure 4.6a shows a CT image through the liver in the arterial phase. The liver contour is slightly irregular, suggesting cirrhotic change. There is a rounded hypervascular lesion in segment 2 of the left lobe of the liver which in the context of a cirrhotic liver suggests a focal hepatoma.
- Figure 4.6b shows large varices in the mesentery.
- Figures 4.6a–c show a large amount of tense ascites in the abdomen and pelvis, in keeping with raised portal venous pressure secondary to alcoholic cirrhosis.
- Figure 4.6d shows that on the scan performed 10 months later there is now a large low-attenuation mass in the left lobe of the liver at the site of the previous hypervascular lesion. The mass has mixed attenuation, predominantly consists of fat, and does not show any hypervascularity on this arterial phase image. The appearances are those of a large fat-containing hepatoma.
- Figures 4.6d and 4.6e show a rounded air-filled structure in the stomach in keeping with a Sengstaken tube to stop a GI haemorrhage from underlying varices. Ascites and varices are again noted.
- Figure 4.6f shows large prevertebral varices heading up towards the gastro-oesophageal junction.

Principal diagnosis

- Alcoholic cirrhosis complicated by a hepatoma in segment 2 which has increased in size and shown fatty degeneration over a period of 10 months.
- Acute GI bleed due to ruptured varices treated with a Sengstaken tube.

Differential diagnosis

- None in this case.

Further management

- GI referral for endoscopic sclerotherapy or variceal ligation.
- Discussion with an interventional radiologist regarding a transjugular intrahepatic portosytemic shunt (TIPSS) if the patient was stabilized.
- Referral to the hepatobilary MDT for further management of the hepatoma if the patient recovers from the acute GI bleed.

Table 4.6a Liver lesions containing fat

Benign	Malignant
• Focal or geographic steatosis	• Hepatocellular carcinoma
• Postoperative packing material (omentum)	• Primary and metastatic liposarcoma
• Adenoma	• Hepatic metastases (rare)
• Focal nodular hyperplasia	
• Lipoma	
• Angiomyolipoma	
• Cystic teratoma	
• Hepatic adrenal rest tumour	
• Pseudolipoma of the Glisson's capsule	
• Xanthomatous lesions in Langerhans cell histiocytosis	

Key points

- Hepatocellular carcinoma is the most common primary hepatic tumour and usually arises in cirrhotic livers secondary to alcoholism or chronic viral hepatitis.
- Other causes include carcinogens, i.e. thorotrast, Wilson's disease, haemochromatosis, α_1-antitrypsin deficiency and tyrosinosis.
- Hepatomas usually present in older patients (sixth to seventh decade) in the West and are more common in males (M:F = 2.5:1).
- Highest incidence is in Africa and Asia, particularly Japan.
- On imaging, hepatomas may be focal and occur more commonly in the right lobe. They may also be multifocal, involving both lobes, or diffuse in appearance.
- Small hepatomas are typically hypervascular on arterial phase scans. Larger tumours tend to appear hypodense because of areas of necrosis.
- The appearance on MRI is variable because of the fat content and extent of necrosis. Fatty change can be seen in up to 35% of small hepatomas.
- Vascular invasion is common, particularly of the portal vein.
- Hepatomas may rupture and cause a massive haemoperitoneum.
- Mortality is high (>90%) with an average survival time of 6 months.
- Treatment is with radiofrequency ablation, intra-arterial chemo-embolization, or surgical resection.

References

Clark HP, Carson WF, Kavanagh PV, Ho CPH, Shen P, Zagoria RJ. Staging and current treatment of hepatocellular carcinoma. *Radiographics* **25**: S3–23, 2005

Federle M, Jeffrey RB, Anne VS. *Diagnostic Imaging: Abdominal.* Amirsys, 2004; 120–3

Prasad SR, Wang H, Rosas H, *et al.* Fat-containing lesions of the liver: radiologic–pathologic correlation. *Radiographics* **25**: 321–31, 2005

Notes

Exam 5

Case 5.1

Clinical details
A 54-year-old female patient presenting with shortness of breath.

Imaging
Figure 5.1a Supine HRCT image of the lungs.
Figures 5.1b–d Prone HRCT images of the lung bases.
Figure 5.1e Plain X-ray of both hands.

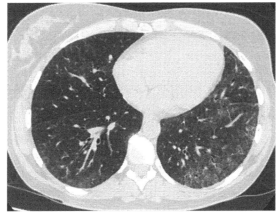

5.1a

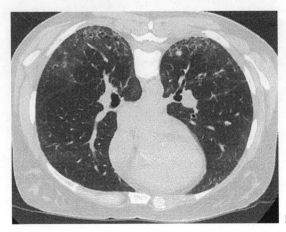

5.1b

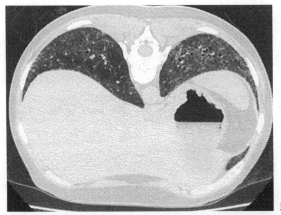

5.1c

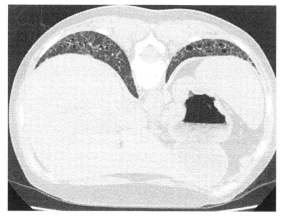

5.1d

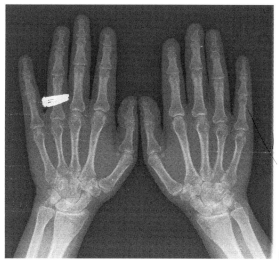

5.1e

Observations and interpretations

- Figure 5.1a shows areas of ground glass shadowing in both lower lobes of the lungs, but more marked on the left. No effusions or cardiomegaly.
- Figures 5.1b–d show that the changes persist at the lung bases with the patient in the prone position.
- There are interstitial infiltrates consisting of areas of ground glass shadowing, septal thickening, and subpleural honeycomb formation, particularly at the left base. The appearances are in keeping with basal fibrosis.
- No oesophageal dilatation or evidence of aspiration pneumonia.
- Figure 5.1e shows resorption of the soft tissues and terminal tufts of the left index, right index, and right middle fingers. No soft tissue calcification, erosive arthropathy, or loss of alignment.

Principal diagnosis

- Scleroderma involvement of the lungs and hands resulting in basal fibrosis and resorption of the terminal tufts of the digits identified above.

Differential diagnosis

- Rheumatoid arthritis—unlikely as there are no features of an erosive arthropathy.

Table 5.1a Differential diagnosis

Causes of basal pulmonary interstitial fibrosis	Causes of acro-osteolysis
• Connective tissue diseases: scleroderma, rheumatoid arthritis • Idiopathic • Asbestosis • Drug-related: amiodarone, bleomycin, busulphan	• Connective tissue diseases: scleroderma, rheumatoid arthritis, psoriasis, dermatomyositis • Trauma: burns, frostbite, electric shock • Absence of pain: diabetes, leprosy, congenital insensitivity to pain • Miscellaneous: porphyria, Raynaud's disease, sarcoidosis, epidermolysis bullosa, hyper-parathyroidism, PVC workers, ergot therapy, multicentric reticulohistocytosis

Further management

- Review any previous chest HRCTs and plain radiographs of the hands to assess progression of basal fibrosis and bone resorption.

Key points

- Scleroderma is a multisystem connective tissue disorder of unknown aetiology affecting several organs and characterized by progressive pulmonary fibrosis.
- The condition is more common in women (M:F = 1:3) and typically occurs between 30 and 50 years of age.
- Pulmonary involvement is seen in 10–25% of patients and manifests clinically as a productive cough and progressive shortness of breath.

- Findings on HRCT scanning include predominantly basal interstitial infiltrates, subpleural honey-combing, and volume loss. There is an increased risk of lung cancer.
- In addition, there may be evidence of air-space shadowing/coarse fibrosis from repeated aspirations secondary to oesophageal dysmotility.
- Involvement of heart muscle can also result in secondary features of heart failure.
- In the absence of heart failure pleural effusions are rarely seen in scleroderma, unlike rheumatoid arthritis where they are a recognized feature.
- Oesophageal involvement occurs in 40–45% of patients. The oesophagus is the first site of involvement in the GI tract. Only the distal two-thirds are affected as the proximal third consists of striated muscle which is not affected. Hypotonia and aperistalsis result in oesophageal dilatation. The lower oesophageal sphincter is patulous, resulting in reflux and potential structuring. There is an increased risk of Barrett oesophagus and adenocarcinoma.
- Musculoskeletal involvement mainly occurs in the hands, with resorption of the soft tissues of the finger tips. Resorption of the distal phalanges or acro-osteolysis is a characteristic feature.
- Soft tissue calcification occurs in the finger tips, elbows, lower legs, ischial tuberosity, axilla, and face.
- An erosive arthropathy in the small joints of the hands can be seen in 25% of patients with soft tissue swelling, periarticular osteoporosis, erosions, and joint space narrowing.
- Erosions occur in other bones: scleroderma is a cause of superior rib notching.
- Remember in the exam—basal fibrosis, dilated oesophagus, and superior rib notching on a chest X-ray = scleroderma!

References

Dähnert W. *Radiology Review Manual* (6th edn). Lippincott–Williams & Wilkins, 2007

Mayberry JP, Primack SL, Müller NL. Thoracic manifestations of systemic autoimmune diseases: radiographic and high-resolution CT findings. *Radiographics* **20**: 1623–35, 2000

Notes

Causes of acreo-osteolysis

Connective tissue disorder
- scleroderma
- RA
- psoriasis
- dermatomyositis

Metabolic
- hyperparathyroidism

Trauma
- burns
- frostbite
- electric shock

Neuropathy
- DM
- leprosy
- congenital insensitivity to pain

Miscellaneous   cleidocranial dysplasia, pyknodystosis
- Raynaud's, sarcoid, porphyria, epidermolysis bullosa,
  hyper-parathyroidism PVC workers
        multicentric reticulohistiocytosis

Case 5.2

Clinical details

A 25-year-old male presenting with epistaxis.

Imaging

Figure 5.2a–b Axial CT nasopharynx, bone windows.
Figure 5.2c Axial T1W MRI nasopharynx pre-contrast.
Figure 5.2d Axial TIW MRI nasopharynx post IV gadolinium.

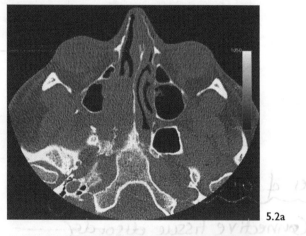

5.2a

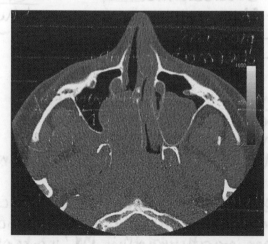

5.2b

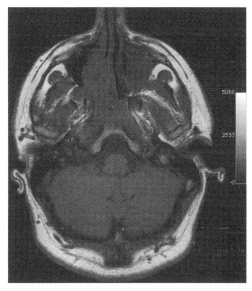

5.2c

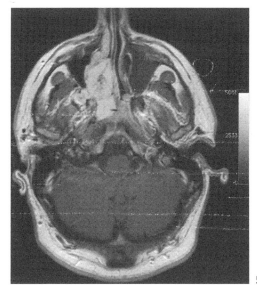

5.2d

Observations and interpretation

- Figures 5.2a and 5.2b show a soft tissue mass in the posterior aspect of the right nasal passage projecting back into the nasopharynx. There is destruction/anterior displacement of the posterior wall of the right maxillary sinus and part of the right pterygoid bone. The mass is expanding the right pterygopalatine fossa.
- Figures 5.2c and 5.2d show that the mass is low signal on the T1W image and enhances intensely post-contrast. There are low-signal flow voids within the mass, indicating a highly vascular lesion. The MRI again shows that the mass is involving and expanding the right pterygopalatine fossa.

Principal diagnosis

- Juvenile angiofibroma.

Differential diagnosis

olfactory neuroblastoma

- The appearances are very typical of a juvenile angiofibroma. Other causes of a nasal mass include an inverted papilloma, lymphoma, sinonasal polyp, haemangioma, lymphangioma, and rhabdomyosarcoma. However, these are all less likely.

↳associated c̄ squamous cell carcinoma.

Further management

- Discussion at specialist MDT.
- Referral for angiography with a view to embolization prior to surgical resection.
- Biopsy contraindicated.

Key points

- Predominantly male patients.
- Mean age at presentation is 15 years.
- The most common benign head and neck tumour.
- Presents with recurrent severe epistaxis and/or nasal obstruction.
- Locally invasive—may extend into the infratemporal fossa, maxillary sinus, sphenoid sinus, or orbit.
- No calcification. *↳superior orbital fissure*
- Arises from the fibrovascular stroma of the nasal wall adjacent to the sphenopalatine foramen.
- Characteristically causes anterior bowing of the posterior wall of the maxillary sinus.
- Vascular supply via internal or external carotid arteries.
- Highly vascular—therefore correct diagnosis is essential to avoid biopsy which could cause a life-threatening haemorrhage.
- Preoperative embolization reduces blood loss at surgery which helps to improve the field of view and enable a more complete resection.
- Recurrence rates may be as high as 40–50% if resection is incomplete.

References

Koh E, Frazzini VI, Kagetsu NJ. Epistaxis: vascular anatomy, origins, and endovascular treatment. *American Journal of Roentgenology* **174**: 845–51, 2000

Laine FJ, Nadel L, Braun IF. CT and MR imaging of the central skull base. Part 2: Pathologic spectrum. *Radiographics* **10**: 797–821, 1990

Momeni AK, Roberts CC, Chew FS. Imaging of chronic and exotic sinonasal disease: review. *American Journal of Roentgenology* **189**: S35–45, 2007

Notes

Angiofibroma

Widening of
-pterygopalatine fossa.

- sphenoid sinus

- inferior orbital fissure [orbit]

- superior orbital fissure [middle cranial fossa]

* Supplied by internal maxillary artery

Case 5.3

Clinical details

A 4-week-old baby presenting with projectile vomiting.

Imaging

Figure 5.3a Sagittal ultrasound image of the upper abdomen.
Figure 5.3b Axial ultrasound image of the upper abdomen.

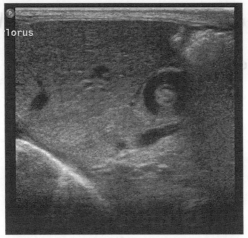

5.3a

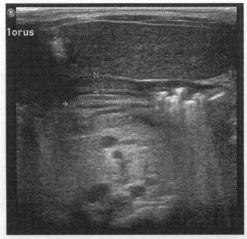

5.3b

Observations and interpretations

- Figure 5.3a shows a transverse view through the pylorus. There is the typical 'target sign' of pyloric stenosis with a ring of hypo-echoic hypertrophied pyloric muscle surrounding the central echo-bright mucosa.
- Figure 5.3b shows a longitudinal view through the pylorus. There is elongation of the pyloric canal to 42.9mm (normally <16mm) and thickening of the pyloric wall to 19mm (normally <3mm).

Principal diagnosis

- Congenital hypertrophic pyloric stenosis.

Differential diagnosis

- None in this case.

Further management

- Barium studies are probably unnecessary because of the classic appearance on ultrasound. The use of ionizing radiation is best avoided if possible.
- Surgical referral.

Key points

- Pyloric stenosis is an idiopathic condition resulting in hyperplasia and hypertrophy of the circular muscles of the pylorus.
- More common in male infants (M:F = 5:1).
- Inherited as a dominant polygenic trait with increased incidence in first-born boys.
- Presents between 2 and 8 weeks of life with non-bilious projectile vomiting. Clinical examination may reveal an olive-shaped mass in the right upper quadrant on palpation.
- Barium studies show elongation and narrowing of the pyloric canal (2-4cm in length). Several signs are described in the literature, including the 'string sign' due to the passage of a small streak of barium through the pyloric canal. There is also gastric distension and hyperperistaltic waves in the stomach, resulting in the 'caterpillar sign'.
- Ultrasound examination typically shows the 'target sign' which is due to a hypo-echoic ring of hypertrophied pyloric muscle surrounding the central echogenic mucosa.
- The diagnosis is made on ultrasound when a single pyloric muscle wall thickness is greater than 3mm and the pyloric canal is longer than 16mm.
- Ultrasound also demonstrates a distended stomach with resting fluid volume and gastric hyperperistalsis.

References

Dähnert W. *Radiology Review Manual* (6th edn). Lippincott–Williams & Wilkins, 2007
Donnelly L (ed). *Diagnostic Imaging: Pediatrics.* Amirysys, 2005
Hernanz-Schulman M. Infantile hypertrophic pyloric stenosis. *Radiology* **227**: 319–31, 2003

Notes

Case 5.4

Clinical details

A 40-year-old male from Peru presenting with a seizure.

Imaging

Figure 5.4a X-ray of left femur.
Figure 5.4b Axial CT of brain pre IV contrast
Figures 5.4c–e Axial CT of brain post IV contrast.
Figure 5.4f Axial T2W MRI of brain.

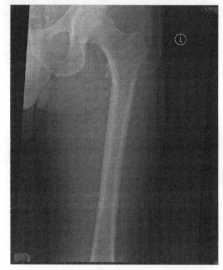

5.4a

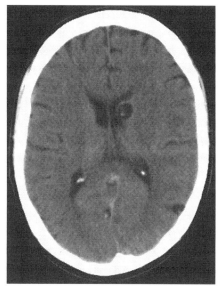

5.4b

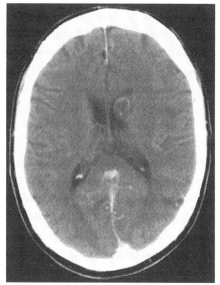

5.4c

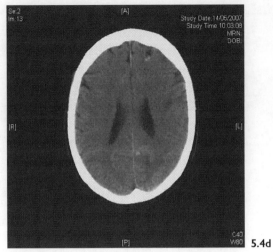

5.4d

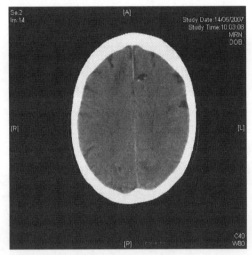

5.4e

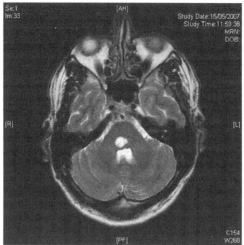

5.4f

Observations and interpretations

- Figure 5.4a shows multiple well-defined 'bullet-shaped' lesions measuring <1cm in the soft tissues of the left thigh. The lesions are calcified with a central lucency and are orientated along multiple muscular planes.
- Figure 5.4b shows a well-defined cystic lesion in the deep white matter adjacent to the anterior horn of the left lateral ventricle. The lesion contains a small calcific focus. Post IV contrast the lesion shows ring enhancement (Figure 5.4c).
- Figures 5.4d and 5.4e show two further lesions in the left frontal lobe measuring approximately 1cm which have thin enhancing walls and eccentric calcified foci, consistent with the scolex of cysticerci.
- Figure 5.4f shows that one of the lesions is adjacent to the fourth ventricle on the T2W image in a subcisternal location. However, there is no obstructing hydrocephalus.
- No significant oedema or mass effect is associated with these lesions.

Principal diagnosis

- Cysticercosis involving CNS and muscles. The lack of associated oedema suggests that the disease is in the chronic phase.

Differential diagnosis

- None
  - ◆ Guinea worm does not cause CNS manifestations and is only endemic in sub-Saharan Africa. It has a coiled appearance of calcification.
  - ◆ Loa loa is only endemic in Central Africa and very rarely has CNS manifestations (after treatment can get meningoencephalitis). The calcifications are a thread-like coils, not bullet-shaped as in this case.
  - ◆ Armillifer has a comma-shaped calcification and does not affect the CNS.

Table 5.4a Differential diagnosis

Curvilinear soft tissue calcification	Ring-enhancing intracerebral lesions
Nerve	Neoplastic
• Leprosy	• Primary tumours—glioma
• Neurofibromatosis	• Metastases
Ligaments	• Lymphoma
• Fluorosis	• Leukaemia
• Diabetes	Infective
• Alkaptonuria	• Abscess
• Tendinitis	• Fungal infections
• Ankylosing spondylitis	• Parasitic – cystercosis
Vascular	Vascular
• Atherosclerosis	• Resolving infarct/haemorrhage
• Aneurysm	• Contusion
• Haemangioma	• Thrombosed aneurysm
• Hyperparathyroidism	Demyelination
Muscles	Radiation necrosis
• Bismuth injections	
• Parasitic infection:	
• cystercicosis (oval)	
• guinea worm (irregular, coiled)	
• loa loa (thread-like)	
• Armillifer (comma-shaped)	
• Myositis ossificans	

Further management

- Compare with any previous imaging if available.
- Refer to infectious disease MDT.
- Immunoserological assay (if not already done).
- Stool for ova culture (if not already done).

Key points

- Cysticercosis is the most common parasitic infection of the CNS worldwide. It is endemic in China, Southeast Asia, India, Latin America, and sub-Saharan Africa.
- Caused by ingestion of the ova of the pork tapeworm (*Taenia solium*) by the faecal–oral route or ingestion of cystercerci in uncooked contaminated pork.
- The shells of ingested larvae dissolve and the embryo is released. The embryo then penetrates the intestinal wall and spreads haematogenously.
- Cysticerci are ovoid parasitic cysts, usually measuring <1.5cm, which contain an invaginated scolex (larval head) bathed in fluid. They can remain dormant for many years. They may degenerate, inducing a granulomatous reaction.
- Imaging features of cysticercosis.
  - ◆ Neurocysticercosis
    - ■ Appearance depends on the stage of the disease: acute phase, single or multiple enhancing lesions with surrounding oedema; chronic phase, well-defined cysts containing a 2–4mm focus of calcification representing the scolex. The end result is multiple calcified granulomas, indicating death of the larvae.
    - ■ They are predominantly located in the brain parenchyma at the grey–white matter interface, and are also seen in the meninges and the spine.
    - ■ Thin-walled mildly enhancing cysts of dimensions 5–20mm are easily seen on CT and MRI (CSF density on CT, ↑T2W, ↓T1W).
    - ■ Intraventricular lesions occur when the larvae are located in a subarachnoid location. This can cause obstructing hydrocephalus, most commonly at the fourth ventricle.
  - ◆ Soft tissue calcification
    - ■ Oval bullet-shaped calcified lesions up to 1cm long with a lucent centre.
    - ■ Orientated along muscle fibres because of compression from surrounding musculature. No compression in CNS; hence they are spherical.

References

Chapman S, Nakielny R. *Aids to Radiological Differential Diagnosis* (5th edn). Saunders, 2009

Dähnert W. *Radiology Review Manual* (6th edn). Lippincott–Williams & Wilkins, 2007

Martinez HR, Rangel-Guerra R, Elizondo G, *et al*. MR imaging in neurocysticercosis: a study of 56 cases. *American Journal of Neuroradiology* **10**: 1011–19, 1989

Noujaim SE, Rossi MD, Rao SK, *et al*. CT and MR imaging of neurocysticercosis. *American Journal of Roentgenology* **173**: 1485–90, 1999

Case 5.5

Clinical details:

A 40-year-old male presenting with weight loss and diabetes mellitus.

Imaging

Figure 5.5a T1W MRI of the liver.
Figures 5.5b–c T1W MRI of the liver post IV gadolinium.

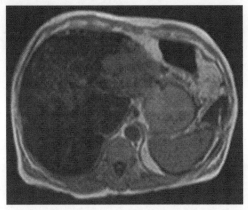

5.5a

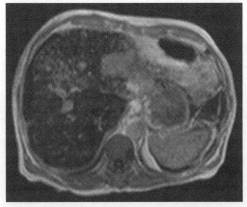

5.5b

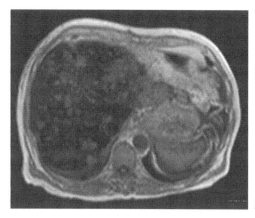

5.5c

Observations and interpretations

- Figure 5.5a shows a large high-signal mass in segment 2a as well as multiple smaller high-signal lesions within the right lobe. The background liver shows diffuse low intensity relative to the spleen, suggesting iron overload. The spleen, pancreas, and bone marrow show normal signal intensity, in keeping with primary haemochromatosis.
- Figures 5.5b and 5.5c show enhancement in the lesions post-gadolinium. The pattern of uptake on a background of low-signal change in the liver suggests multifocal hepatocellular carcinomas.

Principal diagnosis

- Primary haemochromatosis with secondary multifocal hepatocellular carcinomas.

Differential diagnosis

- Multiple liver metastases—however, this would not explain the link with the signal loss in the liver.

Table 5.5a Differential diagnosis

Causes of increased attenuation of the liver on CT precontrast/signal loss on MRI	Causes of a high signal intensity liver lesion on T1W	Association
• Haemochromatosis • Wilson's disease—copper • Colloidal gold treatment • Iodine—amiodarone • Thorotrast • Thallium • Cyclophosphamide • Glycogen storage disease	• Hepatocellular carcinoma • Haemorrhage • Fat deposition • Melanoma metastasis • Contrast agents	• Haemochromatosis complicated by hepatocellular carcinoma

Further management

- Referral to specialist MDT meeting for consideration of palliative chemotherapy. Local treatment such as radioactive microspheres could also be considered.

Key points

- Primary haemochromatosis is a defect in the regulation of iron absorption caused by a genetic disorder.
- Autosomal recessive.
- Accumulation of excess body iron.
- Hepatocytes chelate the excess iron that accumulates, with deposition in the pancreas, heart, pituitary, thyroid, and synovium as well as in the liver.
- Secondary acquired haemochromatosis is due to dietary iron overload or repeated blood transfusions and results in the deposition of iron mainly in the reticuloendothelial system (i.e. spleen and liver).

- If untreated, primary haemochromatosis may progress to cirrhosis, hepatocellular carcinoma, diabetes, cardiac arrhythmias, and congestive heart failure.
- CT features show an increase in the attenuation of the liver of ≥72HU.
- Iron quantification can be performed with MRI. The best sequence is T2* GRE. Relative signal intensity ratios can be uploaded to the website to estimate iron concentration: www.radio.univrennes1.fr/Sources/EN/Hemo

References

Martin DR, Danrad R, Hussain SM. MR imaging of the liver. *Radiologic Clinics of North America* **43**: 861–86, 2005

Queiroz-Andrade M, Blasbalg R, Ortega CD, *et al.* MR imaging findings of iron overload. *Radiographics* **29**: 1575–89, 2009

Notes

Case 5.6

Clinical details

A 30-year-old male patient presenting with diarrhoea, fever, and GI bleeding following a recent holiday abroad.

Imaging

Figure 5.6a Sagittal ultrasound image of the liver.
Figure 5.6b–c Axial CT scans through the liver post IV contrast.

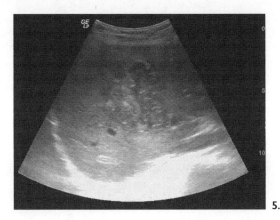

5.6a

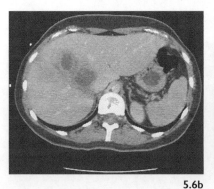

5.6b

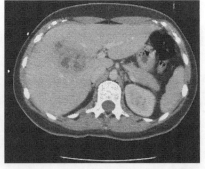

5.6c

Observations and interpretations

- Figure 5.6a shows an area of heterogenous echogenicity in the right lobe of the liver.
- Figures 5.6b and 5.6c show the following.
  - ◆ a multilocular thick-walled cyst seen in segments 5–8 with possible extension into segment 4. There is evidence of enhancement of the wall with no evidence of portal vein thrombosis or gas formation.
  - ◆ There is a low attenuation rim surrounding the mass, in keeping with oedema.
  - ◆ There is no calcification of the wall of the cyst.
  - ◆ The imaged parts of the pancreas, spleen, and left kidney are normal. No daughter cysts are shown in the remainder of the liver.
  - ◆ The underlying liver is normal. There is no evidence of cirrhotic change.
  - ◆ No ascites.

Principal diagnosis

- Given the clinical presentation, the appearances are most likely to be due to an abscess.

Differential diagnosis

- Pyogenic abscess.
- Amoebic abscess.

Table 5.6a Differential diagnosis of adult hepatic cystic lesions

Infective
- Pyogenic/amoebic—history of recent travel
- Hydatid—positive serology, daughter cysts, calcification

Non-neoplastic
- Simple hepatic cysts
- Polycystic liver disease
- Tuberous sclerosis
- Bile duct hamartomas—small lesions with rim enhancement
- Caroli disease
- Pseudocyst—history of pancreatitis
- Haematoma or biloma—history of surgery or trauma

Neoplastic
- Biliary cystadenoma or carcinoma
- Hepatocellular carcinoma, typically solid but may show necrosis
- Cystic metastases: colorectal, ovarian, carcinoid, sarcoma, melanoma

Further management

- Referral to medical microbiology for serum antibody testing is advised.
- Treatment with metronidazole.
- Possible drainage and follow-up CT.

Key points

- Amoebic liver abscess is the most common extra-intestinal manifestation of *Entamoeba histolytica* infection.
- All age groups are affected, but it is 10 times more common in the 20–40-year-old age group.
- Twelve times more common in men than in women.
- Typical imaging appearances are of multiple abscesses with internal septations and nodularity of the walls.
- If left untreated, amoebic liver abscesses can be fatal, with death from sepsis.
- With early diagnosis and treatment with metronidazole alone, mortality has dropped to <1%.
- Aspirates are typically reddish brown—described as 'anchovy paste' or 'chocolate sauce'.
- Ultrasound and CT cannot reliably distinguish between pyogenic infection and amoebic abscess formation.
- Serum antibody detection is an important confirmatory test in the case of amoebic liver abscesses.
- Serological tests are about 90% sensitive for amoebic liver abscess. However, false negatives may arise in the first week and so serial tests are advised.

References

Chavez-Tapia NC, Hernandez-Calleros J, Tellez-Avila FI, Torre A, Uribe M. Image-guided percutaneous procedure plus metronidazole versus metronidazole alone for uncomplicated amoebic liver abscesses. *Cochrane Database of Systematic Reviews* 21 January 2009: CD004886

Mortelé KJ, Ros PR. Cystic focal liver lesions in the adult: differential CT and MR imaging features. *Radiographics* **21**: 895–910, 2001

Mortelé KJ, Segatto E, Ros PR. The infected liver: radiologic–pathologic correlation. *Radiographics* **24**: 937–55, 2004

Notes

Exam 6

Case 6.1

Clinical details

A 70-year-old female patient with weight loss, dyspnoea, and cough. No improvement with antibiotics. No history of immune deficiency.

Imaging

Figure 6.1a Chest X-ray.
Figures 6.1b–c Axial CT images of the lungs post IV contrast on mediastinal and lung windows.
Figure 6.1d Axial HRCT image of the lungs without contrast 2 months after presentation.
Figure 6.1e Chest X-ray 4 months after presentation.

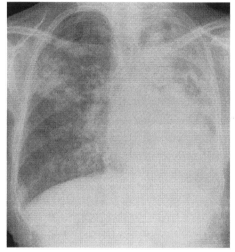

6.1a

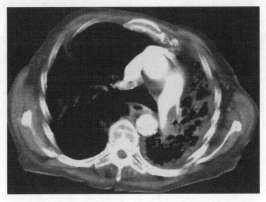

6.1b

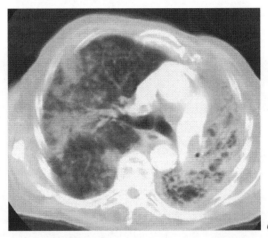

6.1c

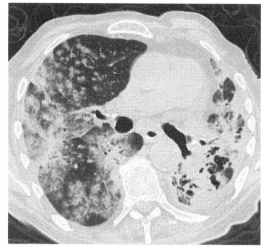

6.1d

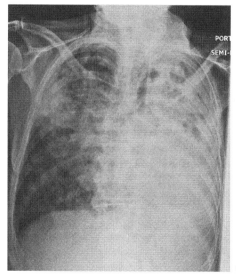

6.1e

Observations and interpretations

- Figure 6.1a shows diffuse bilateral alveolar shadowing. There is global consolidation in the left lung with associated volume loss and consolidation in the right mid-zone. There is nodular opacification involving the right lower zone.
- Figures 6.1b and 6.1c show thrombus in the left main pulmonary artery, marked consolidation and volume loss in the left lung (upper lobe shown), and widespread ground glass centrilobular nodules in the right lung with associated ground glass opacification.
- Figure 6.1d shows volume loss and consolidation in the left lung (lower lobe shown here), a geographical 'crazy-paving' pattern of alveolar ground glass change with smooth septal thickening, and widespread centrilobular ground glass nodules in the right lung (middle and lower lobes shown here). No real change since the CT scan 2 months earlier.
- Figure 6.1e shows that, even allowing for exposure differences, there has been no real change since the original chest X-ray.

Principal diagnosis

- Bronchoalveolar cell carcinoma (BAC).
- Pulmonary embolus left main pulmonary artery.

Differential diagnosis

- Atypical infections—fungal disease (aspergillosis), disseminated pulmonary tuberculosis.
- Aspiration pneumonia.
- Cryptogenic organizing pneumonia.

Further management

- Discussion at MDT meeting.
- Percutaneous lung biopsy of consolidated lung.
- Transbronchial biopsy.

Key points

- Over 50% of patients with localized BAC may be asymptomatic at presentation. Bronchorrhoea (copious watery and 'salty' sputum) is a late symptom and is found in the diffuse variety.
- BAC is associated with smoking and exists in three radiological patterns.
  - Solitary nodule (43%)—subpleural and spiculated due to a desmoplastic or lymphangitic reaction. Tends to be non-mucinous. 'Pseudocavitation' is the presence of bubble-like lucencies caused by tiny air bronchograms. True cavitation is rare. Often produces false negatives on CT/PET.
  - Consolidation (30%) due to growth along alveolar walls and mucin production. The low density of mucin accentuates the 'CT angiogram sign' (clear visualization of vessels in the consolidated lung). 'Crazy-paving' may be seen. These signs are not specific to BAC. The CT angiogram sign may be seen in lobar pneumonia, lymphoma, lipoid pneumonia, infarction, and oedema. The open bronchus sign is seen.
  - Multifocal diffuse disease—multiple ground glass centrilobular nodules 3–5mm in diameter are seen due to the spread of tumour cells to alveolar spaces via the intrapulmonary airways. Occasionally the nodules may reach up to 3cm in size and may be well or poorly defined. Occasional 'tree-in-bud' opacities are seen.
- Nodular opacity with air bronchograms helps to differentiate between BAC and atypical adenomatous hyperplasia.

- Diffuse disease carries a very poor prognosis
- Focal disease (e.g. a solitary spiculated nodule) has a good prognosis if completely resected.

Table 6.1a Causes and features of centrilobular nodules

Causes	Features
Bronchiectasis, bronchiolectasis	Dilated bronchi/bronchioles—'tree-in-bud'
Endobronchial tuberculosis	
Bronchopneumonia	
Bronchiolitis obliterans	Associated with air-trapping
Cryptogenic organizing pneumonia	
Respiratory bronchiolitis	Ground glass nodules
Langerhans cell histiocytosis	Nodules may cavitate
	Sparing of bases (costophrenic region)
Hypersensitivity pneumonitis	Associated with air-trapping
Bronchoalveolar cell carcinoma	Well- or ill-defined nodules

References

Akira M, Atagi S, Kawahara M, Iuchi K, Johkoh T. High-resolution CT findings of diffuse bronchioloalveolar carcinoma in 38 patients. *American Journal of Roentgenology* **173**: 1623–9, 1999

Lee KS, Kim Y, Han J, Ko EJ, ParkC-K, Promack SL. Bronchioloalveolar carcinoma: clinical, histopathologic, and radiologic findings. *Radiographics* **17**: 1345–57, 1997

Oda S, Awai K, Liu D, *et al.* Ground-glass opacities on thin-section helical CT: differentiation between bronchioloalveolar carcinoma and atypical adenomatous hyperplasia. *American Journal of Roentgenology* **190**: 1363–8, 2008

Notes

Case 6.2

Clinical details

A 59-year-old female patient presenting with painless left-sided proptosis and gradual loss of vision in the left eye.

Imaging

Figure 6.2a Axial T1W image of the brain/orbits pre-contrast.
Figure 6.2b Axial fat-saturated image of the brain/orbits post-contrast.
Figures 6.2c–d Axial CT images through the brain/orbits on bone windows.

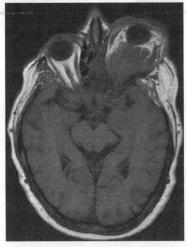

6.2a

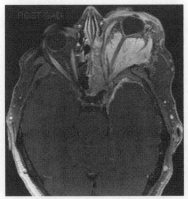

6.2b

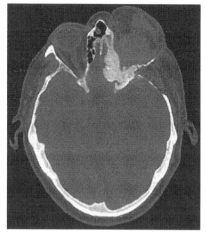

6.2c

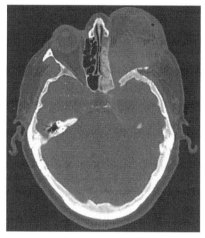

6.2d

Observations and interpretations

- Figure 6.2a shows a low-signal soft tissue mass centred posteriorly in the left retroconal space encasing the optic nerve. The mass is displacing the globe anteriorly, causing the left-sided proptosis.
- Figure 6.2b shows intense enhancement in the mass post intravenous contrast. The mass is involving the left lateral rectus muscle. There is no marked extension of the mass through the optic canal. However, there is contiguous meningeal enhancement around the anterior aspect of the left frontal lobe of the brain. There is opacification of the left ethmoid air cells. The posterior surface of the left globe is tented and there is stretching of the medial rectus muscle and optic nerve.
- Figures 6.2c and 6.2d show sclerosis and expansion in keeping with hyperostosis of the adjacent bones at the left orbital apex and also of the left ethmoid region. Deficient bone along the lateral margin of the left orbit suggests previous surgery/debulking.

Principal diagnosis

- Left optic nerve sheath meningioma with adjacent bony hyperostosis. There is evidence of previous surgery, suggesting that this is recurrent tumour.

Differential diagnosis

- The hyperostosis in this case makes other diagnoses (Table 6.2a) less likely.

Table 6.2a Differential diagnosis of an orbital mass

Causes of an orbital mass	Associated features
Orbital meningioma	• Hyperostosis in adjacent bone • Calcification • 'Tram-tracking' • Perioptic cysts
Optic nerve glioma	• Rarely calcify • No hyperostosis, tram tracking or perioptic cysts
Orbital pseudo-tumour	• Painful proptosis • Not limited to optic nerve
Sarcoidosis	• Similar appearance to pseudotumour • No hyperostosis
Metastasis	• History of malignancy • ± associated bone destruction
Lymphoma Leukaemia	• Not associated with hyperostosis
Schwannoma	• Similar enhancement to meningioma, but no bone changes
Neurofibroma	• Rare
Rhabdomyosarcoma	• Children <10 years
Sarcoma	• Centred on muscle • ± associated bone destruction

Further management

- Review previous imaging to assess progression.
- Suggest referral to specialist head and neck cancer MDT to discuss further treatment options, i.e further surgery versus radiotherapy.

Key points

- Optic nerve sheath meningiomas account for 10% of all intra-orbital neoplasms.
- They are benign tumours but can be locally invasive.
- Female predominance—usually presents in middle age.
- Also seen in young adults with neurofibromatosis.
- Primary orbital meningiomas arise from the arachnoid 'cap' cells in the meningeal layer of the optic nerve sheath or from ectopic rests of arachnoid cells within the orbit.
- 90% of orbital meningiomas are secondary, arising from adjacent structures such as the parasellar region and invading the orbit through the optic canal or superior orbital fissure.
- 95% are unilateral. Bilateral disease is seen with tumour spread across the optic chiasm.
- Presents with progressive loss of visual acuity over several months and painless proptosis.
- Can be tubular, fusiform, or eccentric in appearance.
- Frequently calcified, unlike optic nerve gliomas which rarely calcify.
- Associated with sphenoid wing hyperostosis and perioptic cysts. The latter are dilatations of the nerve sheath containing CSF between the globe and the anterior edge of the meningioma.
- Post IV contrast orbital meningiomas can show the 'tram track' sign of the enhancing tumour surrounding the optic nerve.
- Prognosis—the tumours are slowly progressive with infiltration of the foramina and intracranial structures.
- Surgery is used for debulking or for cosmetic reasons in cases of marked proptosis. Radiotherapy is also used for treatment. Recurrence rates after surgery are high.

References

Mafee MF, Goodwin J, Dorodi S. Optic sheath meningiomas: role of MR imaging. *Radiologic Clinics of North America* **37**: 37–58, 1999

Ortiz O, Schochet SS, Kotzan JM. Radiologic–pathologic correlation: mengioma of the optic sheath nerve. *American Journal of Neuroradiology* **17** 901–6, 1996

Notes

Case 6.3

Clinical details

A 2-year-old boy presenting with abdominal pain.

Imaging

Figure 6.3a Technetium-99m pertechnetate scan.

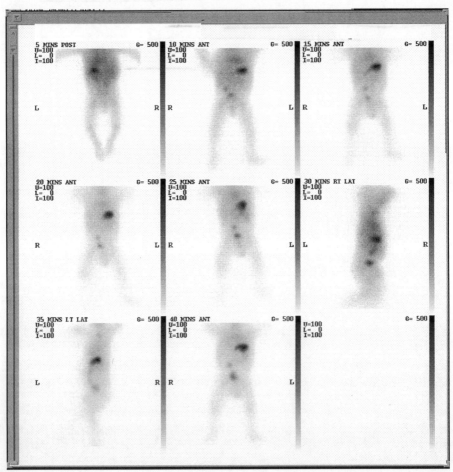

6.3a

Observations and interpretations

- Normal excretion is seen in the region of the stomach and bladder.
- There is a further focal area of excretion in the right lower quadrant of the abdomen just above and to the right of the bladder. This is shown on the 10min image and persists through to the 40min image. It occurs at the same time as excretion in the stomach. This is in keeping with ectopic gastric mucosa in Meckel's diverticulum.

Principal diagnosis

- Meckel's diverticulum.

Differential diagnosis

- Ectopic gastric mucosa in a GI duplication cyst.
- Acute appendicitis.
- GI tract vascular malformation.

Further management

- Referral for a surgical opinion.

Key points

- A Meckel's diverticulum is due to persistence of the vitelline duct which usually closes by the fifth embryonic week.
- 'Rule of 2s'—it occurs in 2% of the population, is usually located within 2 feet of the ileocaecal valve, is approximately 2 inches long, and typically presents before the age of 2 years. M:F = 3:1.
- Usually contains ectopic gastric mucosa, but may also contain pancreatic or colonic mucosa.
- ^{99m}Tc-pertechnetate scan is positive in 90%. ^{99m}Tc-pertechnetate is excreted by mucoid cells of the gastric mucosa.
- Presents clinically with GI tract bleeding due to ulceration, chronic abdominal pain, and intussusception.
- Very rarely malignancies such as carcinoma, sarcoma, or carcinoid can arise within a Meckel's diverticulum.

Table 6.3a Causes of false-positive and false-negative Meckel's scans

Causes of a false-positive scan	Causes of a false-negative scan
• Ectopic gastric mucosa in a gastroenteric duplication cyst, normal small bowel, Barrett oesophagus • Increased blood pool in AVM, haemangioma, hypervascular tumour, aneurysm • Inflammatory conditions: duodenal ulcer, ulcerative colitis, Crohns disease, appendicitis • Laxative abuse • Intussussception, intestinal obstruction, volvulus • Urinary tract obstruction, calyceal diverticulum	• Insufficient ectopic gastric mucosa • Dilution of excreted pertechnetate due to haemorrhage or increased secretions in the bowel lumen • Any cause of rapid bowel transit • Malrotation of the ileum

References

Dähnert W. *Radiology Review Manual* (6th edn). Lippincott–Williams & Wilkins, 2007

Donnelly L (ed). *Diagnostic Imaging: Pediatrics.* Amirysys, 2005

Elsayes KM, Menias CO, Harvin HJ, Francis IR. Imaging manifestation of Meckel's diverticulum. *American Journal of Roentgenology* **189**: 81–8, 2007

Notes

Case 6.4

Clinical details

A 35-year-old male presenting with shortness of breath.

Imaging

Figure 6.4a Chest X-ray.

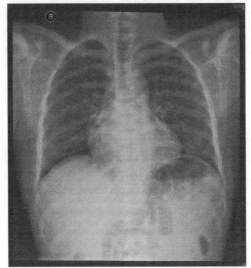

6.4a

Observations and interpretations

- H-shaped vertebral bodies, indicating depression of the central end-plates.
- Cholecystectomy clips in the right upper quadrant.
- High-riding transverse colon, suggesting an absent spleen.
- Generalized sclerosis of the bones.
- 'Snow-capped' sign on the humeral heads in keeping with avascular necrosis.
- Normal heart size—no features of congestive cardiac failure.
- No evidence of acute infection in the lungs.

Principal diagnosis

- Sickle cell disease. The presentation may be due to acute chest syndrome.

Differential diagnosis

- Gaucher's disease. However, this patient does not have splenomegaly.
- Thalassaemia, which can cause sclerosis of the bones and rarely H-shaped vertebrae. However, it does not cause avascular necrosis or gallstones. There is no widening of the medullary space or thinning of the cortices in this case. Thalassaemia may cause hepatosplenomegaly but not autosplenectomy.

Table 6.4a Differential diagnosis

H-shaped vertebrae	Generalized bone sclerosis	Avascular necrosis
• Sickle cell disease • Gaucher's disease • Spherocytosis • Thalassaemia	• Metastases • Myelofibrosis • Mastocytosis • Melorheostosis • Metabolic: hypervitaminosis D, fluorosis, hypothyroidism, phosphorus poisoning • Sickle cell disease • Tuberous sclerosis • Pyknodysostosis, • Paget's disease • Renal osteodystrophy • Osteopetrosis • Fluorosis	• Alcoholism • Sickle cell disease • Steroids • Systemic lupus erythematosus • Gaucher's disease • Pancreatitis • Trauma • Idiopathic • Infection • Caisson disease • Diabetes
	Mnemonic: 5 MS To PROoF	Mnemonic: A SEPTIC E = Erlenmeyer flask deformity (marrow-packing disorders, i.e. Gaucher's disease)

Further management

- Discuss with clinicians as acute chest syndrome can have initially normal chest radiographs (30–60%).
- Supportive treatment—analgesia, rehydration, rest. Consider steroids and antibiotics.

Key points

- Abnormality of haemoglobin (HbS) which results in increased viscosity of the blood under lowered oxygen tension. This results in occlusion of small vessels, infarction, and super-added infection.
- Bones
  - H-shaped vertebrae due to infarction and depression of the central end-plate (~10% of patients).
  - Dactylitis occurs in children under 4 years old and is rarely seen above the age of 7 years. Seen in the diaphysis of small tubular bones (hand–foot syndrome).
  - Avascular necrosis of the femoral and humeral heads.
  - Secondary osteomyelitis. *Salmonella* is five times more common than *Staphylococcus*. One theory is that infarction of the GI tract leads to *Salmonella* bacteraemia, and thus osteomyelitis. Infection is difficult to differentiate from infarction as both give osteopenia and periostitis on the plain film. MRI can help but is also difficult.
  - Haemopoietic marrow replaces fatty marrow—diffuse low-signal change in the bone marrow on T1W imaging.
- Lungs
  - Pneumonia
  - Acute chest syndrome—pulmonary consolidation and some combination of fever, chest pain, and signs of pulmonary compromise. Multiple factors contribute, including pneumonia, fat emboli from bone infarction, hypoxaemia, splinting for rib/sternal infarctions, pulmonary vascular obstruction due to sickling, and endothelial adherence of erythrocytes resulting in infarction of the pulmonary parenchyma. (30–60% of patients have no initial radiographic abnormality.)
  - Chronic pulmonary fibrosis
- Spleen
  - By 5 years of age 94% of sickle cell anaemia patients are asplenic (making patients more susceptible to infection).
  - The spleen becomes small, dense, and calcified over time.
  - Sequestration syndrome—sudden tapping of large amounts of blood in the spleen which can rapidly lead to cardiovascular collapse. Splenomegaly seen on imaging. Rare after 8 years of age.
- Kidneys
  - Renal papillary necrosis.
- Gallstones
  - Pigmented stones—50% of adults and 20% of children.
- Central nervous system
  - Silent or clinically evident stroke.
  - Moyamoya 'puff of smoke' appearance on angiography (reduced blood flow may result in the development of fine collateral vascular channels—present in 35% of sickle cell anaemia patients).

References

Kumar DS, Yadavali R, Concepcion L, Aniq H. Acute chest pain in a young woman with a chronic illness. British Journal of Radiology **81**: 261–3, 2008

Lonergan GJ, Cline DB, Abbondanzo SL. Sickle cell anemia. *Radiographics* **21**: 971–94, 2001

Notes

Case 6.5

Clinical details

A 53-year-old male with hypertensive crises following abdominal trauma.

Imaging

Figure 6.5a Axial T2W MRI image of the upper abdomen.
Figure 6.5b Axial fat-suppressed MRI image of the upper abdomen.
Figure 6.5c Axial 'in-phase' MRI image of the upper abdomen.
Figure 6.5d Axial 'out-of-phase' MRI image of the upper abdomen.
Figure 6.5e Selected axial, coronal, and sagittal ^{123}I-MIBG SPECT images of the upper abdomen (see also Plate 6).

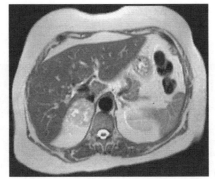

6.5a

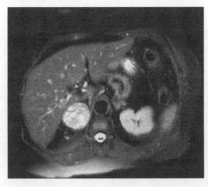

6.5b

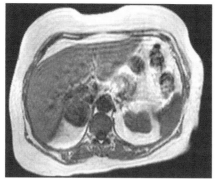

6.5c

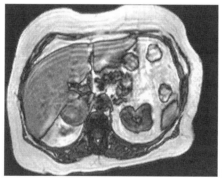

6.5d

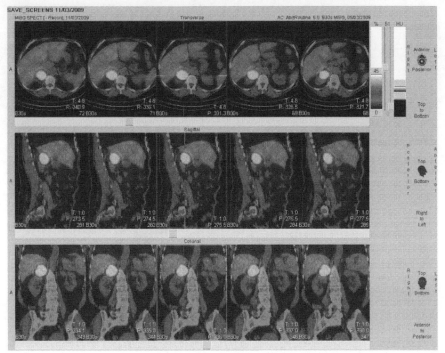

6.5e

Observations and interpretations

- Figures 6.5a–d show a large right adrenal mass which is of high signal on T2W and spectral presaturation by inversion recovery (SPIR) images. There are areas of cystic change within the mass on the T2W images, in keeping with necrosis or haemorrhage. The in-phase and out-of-phase images show no significant signal dropout, indicating that this is not a fat-containing lesion.
- Figure 6.5e shows abnormally increased tracer activity in the right adrenal mass.

Principal diagnosis

- Phaeochromocytoma.

Differential diagnosis

- None in this case because of the increased tracer activity on the MIBG SPECT scan.

Table 6.5a Differential diagnosis of adrenal lesions

Functional adrenal masses	
Adrenal cortex	Adenoma
	Nodular hyperplasia
	Carcinoma
Adrenal medulla	Phaeochromocytoma
	Ganglioneuroma
	Ganglioneuroblastoma
Non-functional adrenal masses	Myelolipoma
	Cyst
	Haematoma
	Hamartoma
	Amyloidosis
	Xanthomatosis
	Neurofibroma
	Teratoma
	Granulomatosis
Metastases	Breast
	Lung
	Lymphoma
	Leukaemia
Pseudo-adrenal masses	Lymph nodes
	Renal
	Splenic
	Pancreas, vessels

Further management

- Check urinary metanephrine and plasma catecholamines: elevated levels of urinary metanephrine or resting plasma catecholamines will support the diagnosis of pheochromocytoma.
- Check family history for conditions associated with pheochromocytoma.
- Referral for surgical resection.

Key points

- On MRI, phaeochromocytomas are typically of high signal intensity on T2W and SPIR imaging.
- Phaeochromocytomas do not contain intracytoplasmic lipid and maintain their signal on opposed-phase gradient-echo images. This lack of dropout of signal intensity differentiates phaeochromocytomas from adrenal adenomas.
- Adrenal adenomas are usually of low signal on T2W images and show loss of signal on the out-of-phase images.
- A hypertensive crisis may be precipitated by abdominal trauma, physical activity, general anaesthesia, or surgical manipulation.
- Phaeochromocytoma has been called the 10% tumour because approximately 10% are bilateral, 10% are malignant, 10% occur in children, and 10% are extra-adrenal (as paragangliomas).
- Extra-adrenal phaeochromocytomas have a higher prevalence of malignancy.
- The most common sites of metastasis include bone, regional lymph nodes, liver, lung, and brain.
- Phaeochromocytomas are associated with other conditions.
  - MEN-2 (autosomal dominant condition)—the prevalence of phaeochromocytoma in MEN-2 is 50% (type 2A) and 90% (type 2B), with unilateral involvement being twice as common as bilateral involvement.
  - von Hippel–Lindau disease (autosomal dominant)—the prevalence of phaeochromocytoma in VHL is 20%.
  - von Recklinghausen neurofibromatosis type 1 (autosomal dominant)—phaeochromocytomas occur more commonly in patients with NF1 than in the general population.
- Non-syndromic familial phaeochromocytoma: some families have a genetic predisposition to develop phaeochromocytoma in isolation without associated conditions.
- Carney's triad: the triad of gastric leiomyosarcoma, pulmonary chondroma, and phaeochromocytoma (most often extra-adrenal and functioning) was first described by Carney in 1977. The cause of the Carney's triad is unknown, and only 58 cases have been reported since its identification in 1977.

References

Benson AB, Myerson RJ, Hoffman J, et al. Pancreatic neuroendocrine GI and adrenal cancers. In: Pazdur R, Coia LR, Hoskins WJ, et al. (eds). Cancer Management: A Multidisciplinary Approach (8th edn). FA Davis, 2004; 273–302

Maurea S, Klain M, Caraco C, Ziviello M, Salvatore M. Diagnostic accuracy of radionuclide imaging using [131]1 nor-cholesterol or meta-iodobenzylguanidine in patients with hypersecreting or non-hypersecreting adrenal tumours. Nuclear Medicine Communications 23: 951–60, 2002

Namimoto T, Yamashita Y, Mitsuzaki K, et al. Adrenal masses: quantification of fat content with double-echo chemical shift in-phase and opposed-phase FLASH MR images for differentiation of adrenal adenomas. Radiology 218: 642–6, 2001

Notes

Case 6.6

Clinical details

A 63-year-old male presenting with acute renal failure.

Imaging

Figure 6.6a–c Axial CT through the kidneys and retroperitoneum without IV contrast.
Figure 6.6d Plain abdominal X-ray.

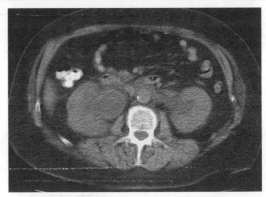

6.6a

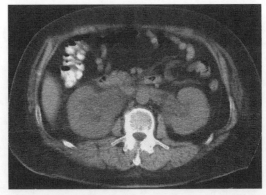

6.6b

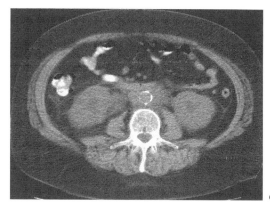

6.6c

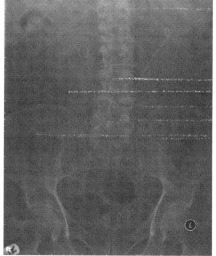

6.6d

Observations and interpretation.

- The scans have been performed without IV contrast because of the history of renal failure.
- Figures 6.6a–6.6c show bilateral hydronephrosis which is more marked on the right. There is soft tissue infiltration around the aorta which is more prominent caudally. The wall of the aorta is calcified; however, the aorta has a normal calibre with no evidence of an aneurysm. No anterior aortic displacement.
- Figure 6.6d shows bilateral ureteric stents *in situ*. Both stents are deviated medially. No other positive findings on this plain film.

Principal diagnosis

- Retroperitoneal fibrosis (RPF).

Differential diagnoses

- Lymphoma (Hodgkin's).
- Metastatic disease.
- Retroperitoneal sarcoma.
- Aortic rupture/retroperitoneal haemorrhage.
- Aortitis.

Further management

- CT of thorax and pelvis to exclude lymphoma.
- CT-guided percutaneous or open retroperitoneal biopsy.
- Trial of steroids/immunosuppressive agents.
- Percutaneous nephrostomy and ureteric stenting.
- Withdrawal of any causative agent such as methysergide treatment.

Key points

- Chronic inflammatory process in the lumbar retroperitoneum/pelvis encasing ureters, IVC, and aorta.
- Primary or idiopathic in 70% of cases, probably due to autoimmune disease. Associated with malignancy in 8% of cases. Peak age is 40–60 years. M:F = 2:1.
- May be associated with drugs—methysergide, β-blockers, hydralazine.
- Associated with other autoimmune conditions such as thyroiditis, rheumatoid arthritis, mediastinal fibrosis, primary biliary cirrhosis, and systemic lupus erythematosus.
- Symptoms are non-specific, ranging from mild back ache to symptoms of acute renal failure as the fibrotic tissue envelops the ureters. Obstructive symptoms due to bowel loop involvement also occur.
- The imaging features include delayed excretion of contrast with unilateral (20%) or bilateral (68%) hydronephrosis, medial deviation of the middle third of the ureters, and narrowing of the ureters at L4/5.
- RPF tends to be located distally at the aortic bifurcation, but can extend cranially to involve the mediastinum and caudally to involve the presacral area.
- In up to a third of cases there is no CT abnormality and the diagnosis is made with surgical biopsy.
- Malignant RPF tends to be of larger volume and to displace the aorta/IVC anteriorly from the spine and the ureters laterally.

- MRI is more sensitive in demonstrating soft tissue in the retroperitoneum without the need for IV contrast agents.
- On CT the soft tissue will enhance if there is active inflammation.
- FDG-PET scanning will demonstrate increased activity whether due to a benign or malignant cause and may be of use in monitoring response to therapy.

References

Cronin CG, Lohan DG, Blake MA, Roche C, McCarthy P, Murphy JM. Retroperitoneal fibrosis: a review of clinical features and imaging findings. *American Journal of Roentgenology* **191**: 423–31, 2008

Vaglio A, Salvarani C, Buzio C. Retroperitoneal fibrosis. *Lancet* **367**: 241–51, 2006

Notes

Exam 7

TNM staging lung Cancer

Tumour

size   T1a ≤ 2cm

            T1b > 2, ≤ 3

            T2a > 3, ≤ 5

            T2b > 5, ≤ 7, visceral pleura

            T3 — > 7 · endobronchial lesion
                     < 2 cm away from the car
                local invasion.
                    chest wall
                    diaphragm
                    parietal pericardium
                    superior sulcur tumour
                    obstructive pneumonitis of the whole lung
                    nodule seperate from same, sa
            T4 nodule in the ~~contralateral~~ lu
                    same lung but not same lob

lymph nodes   N1   peribronchial
                      ipsilateral hilar

                N2 ipsilateral mediastinal
                       subcarinal

                N3 contralateral hilar
                      contralateral mediastinal
                      supraclavicular

     M1a   local thoracic metastatic disease
                    pleural effusions malignant
                    contralateral lung nodules

     M1b   distant or extra-thoracic disease

Case 7.1

Clinical details

A 52-year-old male presenting with haemoptysis and weight loss.

Imaging

Figure 7.1a Coronal FDG PET image of the whole body.
Figure 7.1b Axial fused FDG PET–CT image of the chest (see also Plate 7).
Figure 7.1c Axial fused FDG PET–CT image of the neck (see also Plate 8).

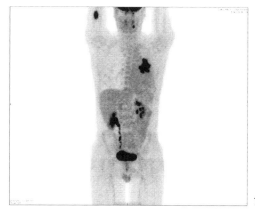

7.1a

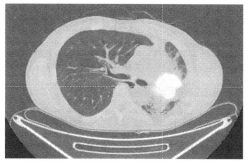

7.1b

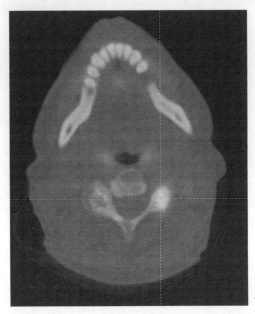

7.1c

Observations and interpretations

- Figures 7.1a and 7.1b show a large FDG-positive soft tissue mass in the left lower lobe of the lung associated with volume loss. The appearances are in keeping with a primary lung tumour.
- Figure 7.1c shows an abnormal FDG focus in the left lateral mass of one of the upper cervical vertebra indicating a skeletal metastasis.
- Figure 7.1a also shows an abnormal FDG focus in the right upper arm suspicious of a metastasis.
- No other abnormal FDG foci are identified. In particular, there is no uptake in the adrenals or in the remainder of the visualized bony skeleton.

Principal diagnosis

- Primary lung tumour with distant skeletal metastases to the right humerus and a cervical vertebra.

Differential diagnosis

- Pulmonary metastasis is less likely—usually multiple and smaller in size.

Further management

- Plain X-rays of the right upper arm to confirm metastasis.
- Discussion at the lung cancer MDT meeting.
- CT-guided lung biopsy.

Key points

- Several studies have demonstrated that PET–CT improves the preoperative staging of non-small-cell lung cancer and reduces the number of futile thoracotomies and the total number of thoracotomies.
- The T stage of primary lung tumours is best assessed by CT and MRI to demonstrate the anatomical extension of the tumour and its relationship to adjacent organs and vessels.
- FDG PET is better than CT or MRI in detecting metastatic lymph nodes which are normal in size by conventional imaging criteria.
- FDG PET is capable of detecting metastases >7mm when CT and MRI are normal or equivocal. A whole-body technique is used to detect metastatic spread. FDG PET is better for lytic metastases. Technetium-99m bone scintigraphy is better for osteoblastic (sclerotic) metastases.
- Patient preparation—the patient is required to fast for 6 hours before a PET scan, during which time he/she should be encouraged to drink only water with no carbohydrates to ensure hydration and promote diuresis.
- The following parameters should be checked as they can affect the image quality/interpretation: history of diabetes, patient weight and height, recent surgery or invasive diagnostic procedures (at least a 4-week interval), radiation therapy (at least a 3-month interval), recent chemotherapy (bone marrow and GI toxicity can vary the biodistribution of FDG as well as tumour uptake), presence of inflammatory conditions (infections, abscesses, tuberculosis, etc.), presence of benign disease with high tissue proliferation (e.g. fibrous dysplasia, sarcoidosis).
- Blood glucose levels should be checked prior to FDG administration and ideally should not exceed 130mg/dl or 7.2mmol/l (except in diabetic patients with higher baseline glucose levels).
- Prior to FDG administration the patient must relax in a waiting room to minimize muscular activity and thereby any physiological uptake of FDG in the muscles. Hyperventilation may cause

uptake in the diaphragm, and stress-induced tension may be seen in the trapezius and paraspinal muscles.

- Head and neck cancer patients in particular should avoid talking or chewing immediately before and after FDG administration to minimize FDG uptake in local muscles (laryngeal and masticatory muscles).
- Patients with brain tumours should wait in a quiet darkened room before (and after) FDG administration.
- Images are acquired 45–60min after injection. Some tumours may require longer uptake period (e.g. neuroendocrine tumours).

Table 7.1a Lung-specific PET indications

Indeterminate lung nodules
Non-small-cell lung cancer • Staging • Monitoring therapy • Restaging • Recurrence
Mesothelioma
Small-cell carcinoma
Radiotherapy planning (can increase the accuracy of delineation of tumour area)

References

Fischer B, Lassen U, Mortensen J, et al. Preoperative staging of lung cancer with combined PET-CT. New England Journal of Medicine **361**: 32–9, 2009

Gurney JW. Determining the likelihood of malignancy in solitary pulmonary nodules with Bayesian analysis. Part I: Theory. Radiology **186** 405–13, 1993

Jemal A, Murray T, Ward E, et al. Cancer statistics, 2005. CA: Cancer Journal for Clinicians **55**: 10–30, 2005

Mack MJ, Hazelrigg SR, Landreneau RJ, Acuff TE. Thoracoscopy for the diagnosis of the indeterminate solitary pulmonary nodule. Annals of Thoracic Surgery **56**: 825–32, 1993

Notes

Case 7.2

Clinical details

A 22-year-old female presenting with right-sided proptosis following a road traffic accident 2 months earlier.

Imaging

Figure 7.2a Axial T2W MRI of the orbits.
Figure 7.2b Coronal T2W MRI of the orbits.
Figure 7.2c Coronal T2W MRI of the cavernous sinus.
Figure 7.2d Coronal T2W MRI of the sphenoid sinus.
Figure 7.2e Selected images from a right internal carotid angiogram—lateral view.

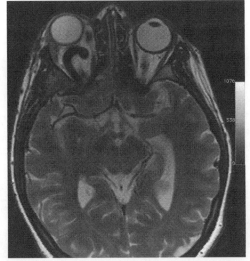

7.2a

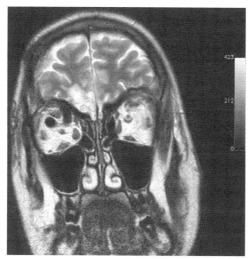

7.2b

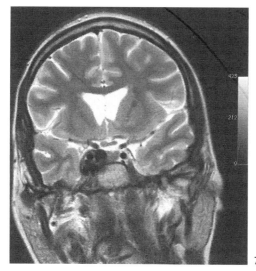

7.2c

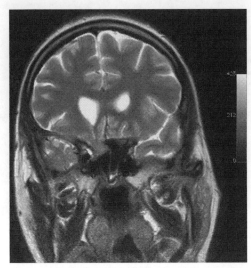

7.2d

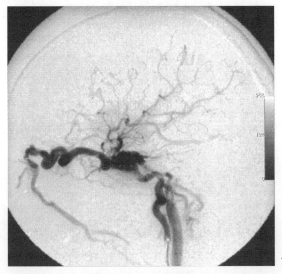

7.2e

Observations and interpretations

- Figures 7.2a and 7.2b show a flow void, in keeping with a dilated vessel in the superior aspect of the right orbit. On the axial image this has a 'hockey stick' appearance, in keeping with a dilated superior ophthalmic vein. There is also right-sided proptosis. The extra-ocular muscles appear normal. On the coronal image there is an area of high signal in the right frontal lobe of the brain, which is likely to represent gliosis and be post-traumatic in nature.
- Figure 7.2c shows dilatation of the horizontal portion of the right intracavernous internal carotid artery. There are further dilated vessels in the right cavernous sinus.
- Figure 7.2d shows an encephalocele with herniation of part of the undersurface of the right cerebral hemisphere into the right sphenoid sinus. In the context of trauma this implies a fracture through the roof of the right sphenoid sinus.
- Figure 7.2e shows early filling of the right cavernous sinus following injection into the right carotid artery. There is communication between the cavernous segment of the internal carotid artery and the cavernous sinus in keeping with a carotid cavernous fistula. There is filling of the superior ophthalmic vein which drains via the facial vein.

Principal diagnosis

- Post-traumatic right carotid cavernous fistula.

Differential diagnosis

- There is no real differential diagnosis in this case.

Further management

- Referral for a neuroradiological opinion for coiling of the fistula.
- Referral for skull base surgical opinion for the encephalocele.

Key points

- The presence of post-traumatic diplopia associated with proptosis and chemosis suggests a diagnosis of carotid cavernous fistula.
- Clinical presentation is with pulsatile exophthalmos, orbital oedema/erythema, reduced vision, glaucoma, headache, deficits of cranial nerves III–VI, orbital bruit, and objective pulsatile tinnitus.
- Carotid cavernous fistula may be spontaneous due to rupture of an aneurysm or secondary to trauma due to a skull base fracture.
- The condition is more common in younger male patients (who are more prone to trauma) and in collagen vascular diseases.
- Usually presents with days or weeks following trauma.
- The fistula results from a tear in the cavernous internal carotid artery which allows arterial blood to enter the cavernous sinus, thereby increasing the sinus pressure and reversing the flow in the venous tributaries.
- Prominent anterior venous drainage results in arterialization of the conjunctiva.
- Findings on unenhanced CT scans of the orbit include a dilated superior ophthalmic vein and cavernous sinus, proptosis, orbital oedema and enlarged extra-ocular muscles.
- On MRI there is enlargement of the cavernous sinus and low-signal flow voids in the dilated veins.

- Isolated dilatation of the superior ophthalmic vein is a potential diagnostic pitfall. This finding has been reported in many other conditions, including cavernous sinus thrombosis, venous varix, and Graves' disease, and as a normal venous variant.
- Angiography is the imaging of choice, with rapid injection to identify the site of the internal carotid artery tear. The cavernous sinus fills rapidly and becomes enlarged after an injection into the ipsilateral internal carotid artery.
- A high-flow fistula develops between the cavernous internal carotid artery and the cavernous sinus.
- The cavernous sinus then drains into the dilated superior and then inferior opthalmic veins, and then into the facial vein.
- Other drainage pathways include via the superior and inferior petrosal sinuses to the internal jugular vein.
- Danger signs on arteriography include filling of cortical veins as these may rupture and result in a subarachnoid haemorrhage.
- Treatment is with either transarterial or transvenous embolization.

References

Gupta S, Biswas R. The hockey-stick sign in a patient with unilateral proptosis. *BMJ Case Reports* 2010: doi:10.1136/bcr.12.2009.2577
Kubal WS. Imaging of orbital trauma. *Radiographics* **28**: 1729–39, 2008

Notes

Case 7.3

Clinical details

A 17-year-old female patient presenting with a lump at the base of the right side of her neck.

Imaging

Figure 7.3a PA chest radiograph.
Figure 7.3b–c Axial CT of the thorax with IV contrast.
Figure 7.3d Coronal CT of the thorax with IV contrast.
Figure 7.3e Axial T1W MRI of the upper mediastinum without gadolinium.
Figure 7.3f Coronal T2W MRI of the upper mediastinum.
Figure 7.3g Axial T1W MRI of the upper mediastinum with gadolinium.

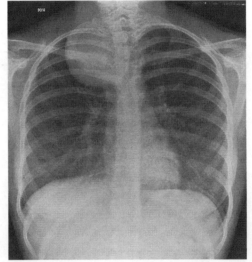

7.3a

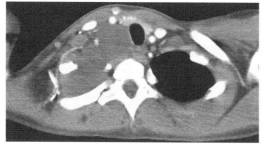

7.3b

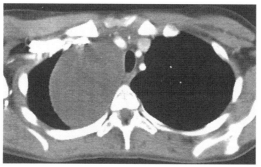

7.3c

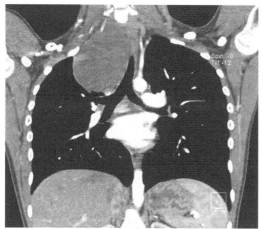

7.3d

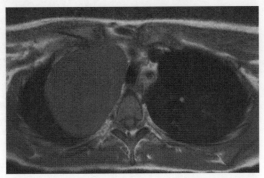

7.3e

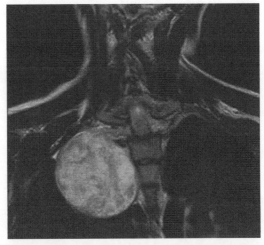

7.3f

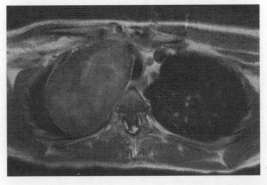

7.3g

Posterior Mediastinal Mass

A. NEOPLASM

- Neurogenic
  @ tumour from the peripheral nerve origin
    ⤷ Schwannoma (only schwann cells)
    ⤷ neurofibroma (all cellular elements)
    ⤷ malignant schwannoma.
  ⓑ sympathetic ganglia origin
    ⤷ ganglioneuroma
    ⤷ ~~go~~neuroblastoma
    ⤷ ganglioneuroblastoma
  ⓒ paraganglia origin
    ⤷ paraganglioma
    ⤷ pheochromocytoma.

- Spinal tumour → metastases
- Lymphoma.
- Thymoma

B. INFECTION → spondylodiscitis

C. VASCULAR MASS → aneurysm

D. TRAUMA → traumatic pseudo meningomyelocele

E. FORE GUT CYST ⎰ bronchogenic
                  ⎱ neuroenteric.
                  ⎲ enteric.

F. OTHER
  ⤷ extra medullary hematopoiesis
  ⤷ lateral meningomyelocele (NF)
  ⤷ pancreatic pseudocyst
  ⤷ loculated pleural effusion

Observations and interpretations

- Figure 7.3a shows a well-circumscribed mass approximately 8cm in diameter arising from the superior mediastinum and extending above the clavicle. There is a sharp interface with adjacent lung. This places the mass in the mediastinum. There is deviation of the trachea to the left side because of its size. No cardiac enlargement. No rib destruction or scalloping. The lungs are otherwise clear.
- Figures 7.3b–d show a non-enhancing mass which is cystic in appearance arising from the posterior/middle mediastinal compartment and extending up to the root of the neck. There is deviation and narrowing of the coronal dimensions of the trachea.
- Figures 7.3e–g show a mass in the superior mediastinum extending to the root of the neck with low signal intensity on T1W and heterogeneously high signal intensity on T2W. There is heterogeneous enhancement on T1W post IV contrast. The enhancement on MRI confirms the presence of solid elements in the mass.
- No direct extension into the neural foramina.

Principal diagnosis

- Neurofibroma (schwannoma).

Differential diagnosis

- Ganglioneuroma and paraganglioma.
- Branchial, bronchogenic, and neurenteric cysts are less likely because of the solid areas in the mass.

Further management

- Surgical excision of mass lesion.
- Biopsy is not recommended—painful and very unlikely to alter management.

Key points

- The actual diagnosis in this case was a schwannoma (nerve sheath tumour).
- The 'cervico-thoracic sign' states that a structure projecting at or above the clavicles, which is effaced superiorly, is an anteriorly placed structure (e.g. a goitre). Conversely, a structure that is clearly demarcated from the lung lateral to it above the clavicles must be situated posterior to the trachea and may lie in the middle or posterior mediastinum.
- The chest radiograph and CT images are suggestive of a cystic lesion as the mass is of uniformly low density and does not exhibit enhancement. However, on MRI there is heterogeneous enhancement with gadolinium, signifying a solid mass lesion.
- Schwannomas are pure connective tissue neoplasms arising from the nerve root sheath. They do not contain nerve cells, unlike neurofibromas which contain both nerve cells and connective tissue elements. Schwannomas are much more common than neurofibromas—together both types comprise the most common cause of benign posterior mediastinal mass lesions. Occasionally they can be malignant.
- 80% of nerve root tumours appear as round masses, and 80% of ganglion tumours appear as vertically elongated masses.
- Nerve root tumours often originate laterally, suggesting that they originate from an intercostal nerve. When there is calcification, this tends to be punctate and involve the mass evenly.
- Neural tumours can be associated with scalloping and separation of ribs (benign slow-growing lesions) and frank invasion (malignant lesions).

- Neural foraminal enlargement is associated with the so-called 'dumb-bell' tumour which arises within the spinal canal and grows outwards.
- The age of the patient is an extremely important clue to the diagnosis of a posterior mediastinal neural mass. Increasing age is associated with more benign pathology.
  - <1 year—neuroblastoma (highly malignant) is the most likely cause. Neuroblastomas are rare after 10 years of age.
  - 1–10 years—ganglioneuroblastoma (intermediate malignancy).
  - 6–15 years—ganglioneuroma (benign).
  - Schwannomas and neurofibromas are rare in children and are most commonly seen after 20 years of age.

Table 7.3a Causes of mediastinal mass lesions

Lesion	Causes
Anterior Loss of heart borders	Thymic lesions Teratodermoid Thyroid 'Terrible' T-cell lymphoma Aortic aneurysm

Middle
  Loss of hila or aortic knuckle
  Oesophageal lesions will extend along the whole length of the mediastinum and may show food debris
	Lymphoma
	Infective lymphadenopathy
	Duplication cysts
	Bronchogenic
	Enteric
	Oesophageal lesions—achalasia, tumours
	Aortic aneurysms
	Pancreatic pseudo-cysts

Posterior
  May extend above the clavicles
  May be associated with rib splaying, scoliosis, or enlarged neural foramina
  Heart borders and hila will be preserved
	Neural
	Nerve root tumours
	Ganglion tumours
	Paragangliomas
	Lateral thoracic meningocele
	Extramedullary haematopoiesis
	Thalassaemia
	Non-neural tumours
	Lymphoma
	Mesenchymal tumours
	Paraspinal abscesses
	Aortic aneurysm

Reference
Whitten CR, Khan S, Munneke GJ, Grubnic S. A diagnostic approach to mediastinal abnormalities. *Radiographics* **27**: 657–71, 2007

Notes

Case 7.4

Clinical details

A 19-year-old male presenting with localized pain in the left lower leg at night.

Imaging

Figure 7.4a Lateral plain X-ray of left lower leg.
Figure 7.4b Selected coronal CT image of left lower leg on bony windows.
Figure 7.4c ^{99m}Tc-MDP bone scan of left lower leg: lateral view.

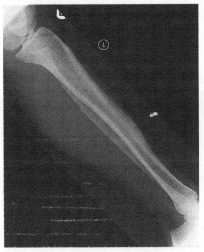
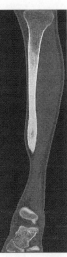

7.4a   7.4b

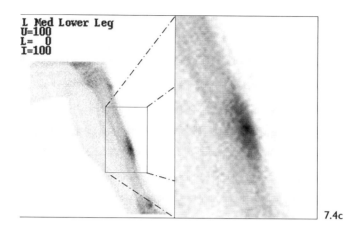

L Med Lower Leg
U=100
L= 0
I=100

7.4c

Observations and interpretations

- Figure 7.4a shows a solid fusiform area of cortical sclerosis at the mid third of the left tibial diaphysis with a central oval radiolucent nidus. There are no malignant features such as soft tissue swelling or aggressive periosteal reaction.
- Figure 7.4b again demonstrates the sclerosis and an underlying central lucent nidus (<1cm in size) on CT.
- Figure 7.4c shows focal increased tracer activity at this site. This image also demonstrates the 'double-density sign', with a small central intense area of increased activity surrounded by more diffuse lesser activity.

Principal diagnosis

- Osteoid osteoma

Differential diagnosis

- Osteoblastoma
- Osteoma
- Osteomyelitis/Brodie's abcess
- Stress fracture

Table 7.4a Differential diagnosis

Causes of a focal sclerotic lesion in the tibia	Appearance on isotope bone scan	Appearance on CT
Osteoid osteoma	Increased uptake	Radiolucent central nidus <1.5cm
Osteoblastoma	Increased uptake	Radiolucent central nidus >2cm
Osteomyelitis	Increased uptake	Linear tract extending to soft tissues
Stress fracture	Increased uptake	Linear radiolucency/fracture
Osteoma	Decreased uptake	No nidus

Further management:

- Discussion at specialist orthopaedic multidisciplinary team meeting (MDT).
- Referral for CT-guided radiofrequency ablation/removal or surgical resection.

Key points

- Strong male predominance (2:1).
- 90% are aged 5–25 years at presentation (average age 19 years).
- May regress spontaneously.
- No malignant potential. Nidus has limited growth potential.
- Localized bone pain which is worse at night and is relieved by non steroidal anti inflammatory drugs (NSAIDS) in 75%. Levels of prostaglandin E_2 are elevated in the central nidus, which causes vasodilatation. The combination of vascular tension and rich nerve supply most likely causes the pain. Aspirin interferes with the synthesis of prostaglandins, thus relieving the symptoms.
- Spinal lesions may present with painful scoliosis.

- Predominantly cortically based in long bones—diaphyseal or metadiaphyseal with >50% located in the femur and tibia. Can be cortical, cancellous, or sub-periosteal in location.
- Other sites include the spine (usually lumbar, typically in the neural arch), hand, or foot.
- Plain radiographs and CT: a smooth central lucent nidus 1.5–2cm in size (>2cm is more suggestive of an osteoblastoma) with dense surrounding osteosclerosis.
- Nuclear medicine: 'double-density sign'. A small area of central increased tracer activity surrounded by more diffuse uptake representing a nidus surrounded by sclerosis. This finding is not specific to osteoid osteoma.
- MRI should be interpreted with the plain film and CT to avoid errors as bone marrow oedema may lead to a misdiagnosis of malignancy. The central nidus is less well visualized than on CT, especially if it is small. MRI is considered better when the lesion is cancellous.
- Angiography: highly vascular nidus has a blush in the early arterial phase which persists in the venous phase.
- Treatment consists of percutaneous radiofrequency ablation and ethanol, laser, or thermocoagulation therapy under CT guidance.

References

Assoun J, Richardi G, Railhac JJ, et al. Osteoid osteoma: MR imaging versus CT. Radiology **191**: 217–23, 1994

Helms CA, Hattner RS, VoglerJB. Osteoid osteoma: radionuclide diagnosis. Radiology **151**: 779–84, 1984

Notes

Case 7.5

Clinical details

A 17-year-old with a previous history of seizures presenting with abdominal pain and macroscopic haematuria.

Imaging

Figures 7.5a–b Selected axial CT images of the abdomen in the portal venous phase.

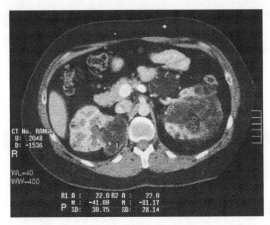

7.5a

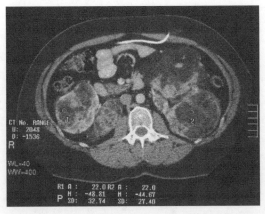

7.5b

Observations and interpretations

- Figures 7.5a and 7.5b show bilateral renal masses >4cm in size containing predominantly fat (region of interest, ~ −40 to −80HU). There is no infiltration of the peri-renal or hilar fat.
- No radiological signs of active haemorrhage.
- There is tubing in the subcutaneous tissue extending into the peritoneum consistent with a ventriculoperitoneal shunt.

Principal diagnosis

- Tuberous sclerosis—bilateral angiomyolipomas and ventriculoperitoneal shunt most likely secondary to giant cell astrocytoma causing obstructive hydrocephalus.

Differential diagnosis

- None in this case

Further management

- Referral to urologist for management of the acute haematuria.
- Consideration of angiography and embolization if an active bleeding site is demonstrated in one of the angiomyolipomas.
- Suggest genetic counselling, if not already undertaken, as this is autosomal dominant with incomplete penetrance.

Key points

- Tuberous sclerosis is a rare condition (1 in 12000). Inheritance is autosomal dominant with incomplete penetrance. It is a neurocutaneous syndrome with benign congenital hamartomatous tumours in multiple organs.
- The classical clinical presentation is with Vogt's triad of epilepsy, mental retardation (half have normal intelligence), and adenoma sebaceum.
- Neurological involvement includes cortical tubers or subependymal nodules (in 95%), subependymal giant cell astrocytomas (typical location is in the foramen of Monro, which commonly leads to obstructive hydrocephalus), and white matter lesions.
- Cardiac involvement occurs with cardiac rhabdomyomas: 75% of these occur before the age of 1 year. Spontaneous regression can occur in 70% of children by 4 years of age.
- Pulmonary and thoracic involvement is seen with lymphangioleiomyomatosis. The typical finding on CT is multiple thin-walled cysts of variable sizes. Can have recurrent pneumothorax and chylous pleural effusions.
- Renal involvement is characterized by angiomyolipomas. Renal cysts, renal cell carcinomas, and oncocytomas can also occur.
- Angiomyolipomas are benign tumours composed of blood vessels, smooth muscle cells, and fat cells. When associated with tuberous sclerosis they tend to be large bilateral lesions. When the lesions reach a size >4cm they are usually treated surgically because of the risk of haemorrhage.
- GI involvement includes polyps, intestinal leiomyomas, hepatic harmatomas, lipomas, angiomyolipomas, and fibromas.

Reference

Umeoka S, Koyama T, Miki Y, Akai M, Tsutsui K, Togashi K. Pictorial review of tuberous sclerosis in various organs. *Radiographics* 28: doi:10:1148/rg.e32, 2008

Notes

Case 7.6

Clinical details

A 55-year-old male patient with a chronic illness presenting with worsening renal function.

Imaging

Figures 7.6a–c Axial CT scans through the abdomen/pelvis, unenhanced.

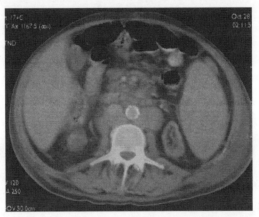

7.6a

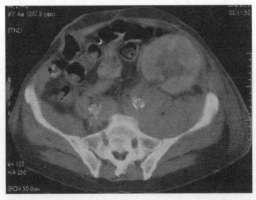

7.6b

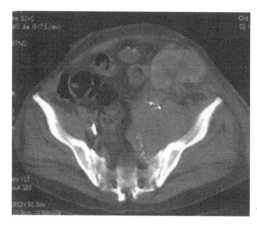

7.6c

Observations and interpretations

- Figure 7.6a shows the following.
  - ◆ Splenomegaly.
  - ◆ Atrophic native kidneys.
  - ◆ Retroperitoneal lymphadenopathy in the aortocaval and para-aortic regions as well as along the route of the small bowel mesentery.
- Figures 7.6b and 7.6c show the following.
  - ◆ A transplanted kidney in the left iliac fossa with moderate dilatation of the renal pelvis.
  - ◆ A large soft tissue mass in the left side of the pelvis involving the left iliopsoas muscle in keeping with further lymphadenopathy. The mass is encasing the left external iliac artery and is situated posterior to the transplanted kidney in the region of the anastomosis/surgical clips.
  - ◆ Small-volume lymphadenopathy medial to the right external iliac artery.
  - ◆ Heavy calcification of the iliac vessels, which can be a feature of renal osteodystrophy.

Principal diagnosis

- Obstruction of renal transplant due to post-transplant lymphoproliferative disorder secondary to immunosuppressive treatment.

Differential diagnosis

- None in this case.

Further management

- Biopsy of lymph node mass to confirm histological subtype.
- Referral and discussion at specialist lymphoma/renal MDTs with a view to further treatment for lymphoma and management of renal transplant.

Key points

- The incidence of malignant neoplasms is increased in renal transplant patients, with the most common being renal cell carcinoma, Kaposi's sarcoma, and lymphoma.
- Lymphoma in transplant patients shows aggressive atypical features unlike the lymphomas that occur in the general population.
- These lymphomas are almost always fatal if untreated.
- If detected early and treated by reduction of the immunosuppressive agents, most cases will resolve.
- The dose threshold for an immunosuppressive drug causing post-transplant lymphoproliferative disorder (PTLD) has not been established.
- Most transplant patients who develop lymphoma are actively infected with Epstein–Barr virus.
- In immunocompromised patients weak or suppressed T-cell function leads to an excessive B-cell proliferation which results in a disease spectrum ranging from mild diffuse polyclonal adenopathy to malignant monoclonal lymphoma.
- Most lymphomas in immunocompromised patients are of the B-cell non-Hodgkin's type, although Hodgkin's, Burkitt's, and T-cell lymphomas have been reported.
- The incidence of malignancies in organ transplant patients is ~6%, and PTLD accounts for 20% of the tumours.

- PTLD occurs as early as 1 month after transplantation. If azathioprine is the immunosuppressant medication taken, the average length of time to develop PTLD is 48 months, whereas with cyclosporine it is 15 months.
- Reduction of immunosuppression is the major form of therapy for PTLD. Acyclovir, an antiviral agent, can be given to treat the Epstein–Barr virus infection.
- Extranodal disease (81%) is more common than lymphadenopathy (22%) in patients with PTLD. Single or multiple organ masses are the characteristic radiographic presentations of PTLD. Any of the solid organs, hollow viscera, abdominal, retroperitoneal, and iliac lymph nodes, retroperitoneal musculature, or peritoneum of the abdomen can be involved in PTLD.
- The transplanted renal pelvis/anastomosis is the most common site of involvement by lymphoma.

Table 7.6a Post renal transplant complications

Peri-renal and renal fluid collections
- Haematoma
- Lymphocele
- Seroma
- Abscess
- Urinoma

Vascular complications
- Renal artery stenosis
- Iliac artery stenosis
- Renal artery thrombosis
- Intra-renal arteriovenous fistula and pseudo-aneurysm
- Extra-renal pseudo-aneurysm
- Renal graft torsion
- Renal vein thrombosis

Ureteric obstruction

Post-transplant malignancies
- Lymphoma
- Kaposi's sarcoma
- Renal cell carcinoma
- Acute and chronic rejection

References

Sebastià C, Quiroga S, Boyé R, Cantarell C, Fernandez-Planas M, Alvarez A. Helical CT in renal transplantation: normal findings and early and late complications. *Radiographics* **21**: 1103–17, 2001

Vrachliotis TG, Vaswani KK, Davies EA, Elkhammas EA, Bennett WF, Bova JG. CT findings in post-transplantation lymphoproliferative disorder of renal transplants. *American Journal of Roentgenology* **175**: 183–8, 2000

Notes

Appendix
Checklist for rapid reporting

Chest X-ray

Bones

- Rib fractures
- Missing rib/rib lesion
- Fractured humeral head
- Fractured clavicle
- Destroyed pedicle
- Rib notching—coarctation
- Look at cervical spine—injuries or bony destruction

Lungs

- Mastectomy
- Neck masses—soft tissue mass lesions
- Air space shadowing
- Mass—review apices and behind the heart. Masses are sometimes projected beneath the diaphragmatic silhouette. Look for a mass lesion adjacent to the aortic knuckle.
- Pulmonary metastases
- Pneumothorax
- Lobar collapse
- Cavity

Mediastinum

- Pneumomediastinum
- Pericardial effusion
- Hilar lymphadenopathy/mass
- Coarctation
- Dilated oesophagus
- Mediastinal mass

Pleural space

- Pleural mass
- Pleural effusion

Abdomen/lumbar spine/pelvis X-ray

Bowel

- Small/large bowel obstruction
- Perforation
- Thumb printing in colon
- Pneumatosis intestinalis
- Ascites—central bowel loops
- Inguinal hernia

Solid organs

- Hepato/splenomegaly
- Enlarged renal outlines
- Gas in bladder lumen
- Emphysematous cystitis/cholecystitis
- Pelvic mass
- Calcified pancreas, liver, etc

Bones

- Sacro-iliitis
- Missing pedicle
- Discitis
- Burst fracture of lumbar spine
- Pelvic fracture
- Lytic lesion in pelvis
- Fractured femoral neck
- Avascular necrosis of femoral heads

Calcifications

- Renal stones
- Ureteric stones
- Gallstones
- Porcelain gall bladder
- Chronic pancreatitis
- Bladder calculi
- Pelvic dermoid
- Calcified liver—mass or parenchymal

Shoulder X-ray

- Anterior dislocation
- Posterior dislocation
- Acromioclavicular joint disruption
- Fracture/avascular necrosis of humeral head
- Pulmonary metastases
- Mass at lung apex
- Missing rib, fracture of rib
- Pneumothorax

Foot/ankle X-ray

- Base of fifth metatarsal fracture
- Lisfranc injury
- Look for minimally displaced oblique fractures of the lateral malleolus on the lateral view.
- Osteonecrosis of tarsal bones

Wrist X-ray

- Scaphoid fracture
- Lunate/perilunate dislocation
- Scapholunate dissociation
- Impacted radial fracture

- Buckle fracture—child
- Torus fracture—child
- Salter–Harris fracture—child
- Triquetral fracture: lateral view—bone fragment posterior to carpus
- Hamate fracture
- Osteonecrosis of carpal bones

Knee X-ray

- Lipohaemarthrosis
- Osteochondral defect
- Tibial plateau fracture
- Segond fracture

Skull/cervical spine X-ray

- Air in orbit
- Intracranial air
- Depressed skull fracture
- Linear skull fracture
- Air/fluid level in sphenoid sinus
- Odontoid peg fracture
- Hangman's fracture
- Pre-vertebral soft tissue swelling—injury or infection

DO NOT FORGET TO LOOK AT THE EDGES OF THE FILM!

Index

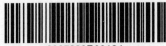

Printed in Great Britain
by Amazon.co.uk, Ltd.,
Marston Gate.